The A List

9 Guiding Principles for Healthy Eating and Positive Living

NEW EDITION

*To Karen,
Wishing you
Continued health
& happiness!
Roslyn Franken*

Roslyn Franken, MA HSI

The A List: 9 Guiding Principles
for Healthy Eating and Positive Living
NEW EDITION

By Roslyn Franken
For permission to reproduce any part of this publication, or to book the author for speaking engagements, media appearances or private counseling, call **1.877.852.5852** or send email to **info@roslynfranken.com**

Visit Roslyn Franken online at **www.roslynfranken.com**

Published by 10-Q Publishing
Ottawa, Ontario, Canada
www.10QPublishing.com
info@10QPublishing.com

Printed and bound in Canada

The advice and recommendations in this book are the opinion of the author and should in no way replace the services of a qualified medical professional. Care has been taken to appropriately reference any books or quotations used in the writing of this book. The author and publisher welcome any information enabling them to rectify any references or credit in subsequent editions.

First published by Book Coach Press, Ottawa, Ontario, Canada, 2006.
ISBN 0-9739071-5-0, © 2006 Roslyn Franken

Cover photography © Photographer: Scott Rothstein | Agency: Dreamstime.com

Library and Archives Canada Cataloguing in Publication

Franken, Roslyn, 1965-
     The A List: 9 Guiding Principles for Healthy Eating and Positive Living / Roslyn Franken.

Includes bibliographical references.
ISBN 978-0-9784274-0-5

     1. Health. 2. Nutrition. 3. Conduct of life. I. Title.

RA776.5.F74 2007   613   C2007-906405-1

Table of Contents

Acknowledgements

There are a few very special people who I want to acknowledge, for without their inspiration and continued support, I would not have written the book you're about to read. The first is my mother, Sonja Franken. She died on January 14, 2004, of primary peritoneal cancer. She survived a remarkable and courageous twenty-three year battle, surpassing all of her doctors' expectations. Given her type of cancer and condition upon diagnosis, her life expectancy was no more than two years. Yes, my mother was a survivor in the truest sense of the word. As a young teenager, she survived the concentration camps of Nazi Germany, where she lost her parents, two brothers, and a sister. When she got news of her cancer, she told the doctor, *"Hitler didn't get me, and neither will my cancer." "I have too much to live for,"* she used to say. Her determination, will to live, and relentless courage are an inspiration to me and all who knew her. To my mother I say, *"Thank you, mama, for teaching me what it means to be resilient in the face of whatever adversity is thrown my way, no matter what challenges must be faced, or what painful losses must be endured. Thank you, mama, for always believing in me. Thank you for everything you've given me to live a healthy, happy and meaningful life. Your example is, and will always be, a powerful force I know I can depend on."*

The next very special person I am so very proud to acknowledge is my father, John Franken. He is now 85 years old and still going strong. He, too, is a survivor in the truest sense of the word. While my mother was enduring the war-time atrocities in Europe, my father was fighting for his survival on the other side of the world in Japan. He survived the Japanese slave labour camps as a prisoner of war. For years he, like my mother, never knew from one day to the next if he would see another tomorrow. Yet despite the horrific experiences of his youth, my father is one of the most positive, humble, thoughtful and generous of spirit people you could ever meet. His strong spiritual beliefs that everything in life is meant to be, that there are no coincidences, and one must always recognize and give thanks for one's blessings are, I believe, what continue to drive him from one day to the next filled with hope, acceptance and determination. *"Thank you, papa, for all the spiritual wisdoms and moral values you have taught me. Thank you for always believing in me. Thank you for everything you have given me to live a healthy, happy and meaningful life. Your example is, and will always be, a powerful force I know I can depend on."*

Another very special person I would like to acknowledge is my husband, Elliott Smith, professional magician and co-author of *Highway to Success: The Entertainer's Roadmap to Business*. Needless to say, I am his biggest fan. The most amazing magic he performs is not necessarily what you see on stage, but rather in the magic he brings into my life on a day-to-day basis. When he puts his mind to something, he knows no limits or boundaries. He creates things in his imagination, and then magically turns them into reality. This is truly one of his many gifts. To Elliott I say, *"Thank you for your love, affection and support in whatever I choose to do. Thank you for teaching me to believe in myself, to visualize my dreams, and turn them into reality. This book is living proof. Thank you for all that you give me and all that we share. Your example is, and always will be, a powerful force I know I can depend on."*

Lastly, I would like to acknowledge two very special people, Dianne Villeneuve Labonté, business owner and Dr. Vic Weatherall, chiropractor. What makes these individuals special is the personal integrity they bring to their respective businesses, and their genuine desire to make a difference in people's lives through increased health and wellness. To Dianne and Vic I say, *"Thank you for always being there with unfailing encouragement and support, especially in the early days of building my counseling practice. It is greatly appreciated."*

In addition, I would like to thank every client who has put his or her faith and trust in me and my counseling program. To my clients I say, *"Thank you for your commitment to improving your health and changing your lives for the better. You have been, and continue to be, an endless source of inspiration and learning for me, both professionally and personally."*

Introduction

If you're like many others who struggle with food, weight and lifestyle issues, you've probably tried all kinds of restrictive diets and schemes that promise fast and easy results. How have these worked for you so far? My guess is that you're here right now because these methods failed you, leaving you feeling even more discouraged than when you started. Like countless others, you ended up going back to your old eating and lifestyle habits, and put on even more weight as a result. However, I know you're also here now because you're not ready to give up. This is a sign of great strength and courage, for which I offer you my heartfelt congratulations. Just by coming this far, you've already proven that you want a sustainable solution that will finally get you the long-term healthy eating, positive living and weight control results you so desire for a life of greater health and happiness.

From my own and others' experiences, I've come to the conclusion that going on and off rigid diets and programs is just as hard on you mentally, emotionally and spiritually, as it is physically. Every time you start anew, you set out with the best of intentions, full of hopes and dreams, believing that this time you have found the magic answer. So why isn't it working? The answer is simple. FAD DIETS, GIMMICKS AND QUICK FIX SCHEMES DON'T WORK LONG-TERM!

How do I know all this, you ask? I know because not only have I proudly triumphed over my own battles with food and weight, but I have also helped many others overcome their similar challenges. As an author, counselor, and professional speaker, I specialize in helping people learn to eat better, feel better and live better through my 9 guiding principles for healthy eating and positive living. My mission is to help people just like you to reprogram their relationship with food and their inner selves for enhanced self-image, greater health and improved quality of life. Most of the people I help are women. However, in many cases, the men and children in their lives will adopt the same changes, and in turn create greater health and happiness for themselves. All this is to say, that men and children can equally benefit from the information and insights presented herein.

I do not make false promises or guarantees that you'll reach your healthy weight as quickly and easily as you'd like. What I do promise is to help you gain the necessary insights into your behaviours and attitudes toward food, exercise and your inner-self to eat better, control your weight, and enjoy the power of positive living for life, in the healthiest, most practical and sustainable way possible. This means without going hungry or feeling deprived.

As a cancer survivor, I already know and understand what it means to lose your health, which is why helping others improve their health is so important to me. I don't know whether or not my cancer will ever come back, but what I do know is that I can do everything within my power and control to minimize the risks of cancer, or any other disease, for that matter, by being good to my body, mind and soul through the practices of healthy eating and positive living.

Overcoming cancer at age thirty forced me to start a journey of self-reflection, and search for meaning and purpose in my life. I yearned to understand myself, others and the world around me in a much deeper and more meaningful way. Through this process, I learned that my life's purpose is to help others in their process of self-discovery, and their own personal search for meaning and life satisfaction. What I've concluded from my ongoing journey, is that we all have choices in every thought we have, belief we hold and action we take. I learned that we create our own realities based on how we view ourselves, others and the world in which we operate.

Therefore, you may gauge your success simply by the number on the scale or size of your clothes, but believe me when I say that it goes so much deeper than these superficial measures. Your success will be seen and felt in your brighter eyes, happier disposition, the extra bounce in your step, and a greater joie de vivre. It will all culminate in your greater sense of self, improved health and more positive view of yourself, your life, and those around you. That's what it's all about. Along with guidance, tools and techniques, I will give you the positive inspiration and encouragement you need to turn your health and quality of life around.

Before I continue, I want to thank you for putting your trust and faith in the guidance and support that I am offering you through the experiences and perspectives covered in this book. My intent is to inspire, motivate and help you see that a lifetime of healthy eating and positive living for improved weight control and quality of life ARE truly possible. My wish is for you to learn that not only is it completely feasible to achieve long-term results WITHOUT diets, pills, going hungry or feeling deprived, but that with some proper guidance and support, you CAN do it and WILL do it, too.

This book gives you the guiding principles that will empower you to become the next courageous person who takes control of their health and weight for lifelong results. On the first stop of our journey, we'll look at how the world around us influences our eating and lifestyle habits. At the next stop, we'll look at what is required to rise above those influences, and take back control of our health and quality of life. The remainder of our journey together will focus on my "A" list, including the 9 guiding principles for healthy eating and positive living for maximized health and happiness.

The A List's 9 guiding principles are as follows:

1) *Ambition*   6) *Assessment*

2) *Attitude*   7) *Accountability*

3) *Attainability*   8) *Appreciation*

4) *Awareness*   9) *Acceptance*

5) *Activity*

What You'll Need

Throughout this book, there will be questions for you to answer. I have provided some space, but you may find that you need more. I ask that you keep a journal or blank paper at your side to jot down any extra thoughts that come to mind. I suggest revisiting these questions on a regular basis, perhaps monthly to start, and write down your replies as if it's the first time you're answering them. You may find over time that your responses will change. Keep copies of all your notes and answers. Jot down your own questions as they come to mind.

When you answer the questions, be sure to sit in a quiet place with no distractions. Breathe. Relax. Try not to judge your answers. Let the ideas flow. Write whatever thoughts come to mind in response to the questions.

At other points in the book, such as when I teach you about food-awareness, you may wish to have a calculator handy, as some simple calculations will be required.

What to Expect

Will this be an easy ride? Not necessarily. There may be unexpected bumps and turns along the road, but with focus and determination to settle in at your final destination, know that you can always get yourself back on track. For some it will be easier than others, as you are asked to stretch beyond your self-limitations. You will be asked to release yourself from the negative thinking traps keeping you stuck and powerless. You will be asked to look at yourself in the mirror and see beyond the outer shell, to get to know the real person who lies within.

My book is not like others, in that it does not offer a superficial and temporary solution as with typical diet approaches. For lifelong results, you need to dig deep and uncover the true, underlying issues that are contributing to your ongoing food, weight and lifestyle problems. If this sounds a bit daunting, please take comfort in knowing that you do not have to do it alone. I will act as your guide to help you break through the barriers that have been holding you back till now. I'll also teach you how to find and reach out for the proper support you need. Let the ideas and perspectives provoke you to think in new ways, expand your realm of what is possible, inspire your self-confidence, and motivate you into positive action. Are you ready? Then all aboard! We're off to a wonderful destination of healthy eating and positive living for improved weight control and quality of life.

DISCLAIMER: The information and opinions shared in this book are not to replace medical advice. It is strongly recommended that readers consult with their doctors prior to making any changes to their regular diet and lifestyle, whether for the purpose of weight management and control, or any other health or medical related reasons. The information and opinions expressed herein are to be used for educational purposes only and at the reader's own discretion. Results are not guaranteed and will vary from person to person depending on individual medical status, age, gender, level of effort and other related health factors.

The Ripple Effect

How the World We Live In Impacts Our Health and Eating Habits

Fast-paced and Ever-changing

We live in a world so fast-paced and ever-changing, that for many of us, life feels like just one long To-Do list. We're so busy jumping from task to task, trying to solve problems, take care of others, and get things *"done"*, that we're completely losing touch with who we truly are, and what is truly meaningful and important to us. To keep up with all the pressures and demands of daily life, we've become so stressed and overwhelmed that it's costing us our health. We are paying for it with poor eating habits, insufficient physical activity, and too little proper rest and down time to have real fun, spend time with our family and friends, or just *"be"*. When I say health, I don't just mean our physical health. I'm talking about our mental, emotional and spiritual health as well. The problem is we are not machines. We are humans, yet the way we interact with each other, it is sometimes almost easier to deny our humanness. As a result, we often find ourselves overtired, and perhaps dissatisfied in our work, unhappy in our relationships and/or facing financial distress, leaving us with a sense of emptiness and powerlessness at the end of the day.

Many of us go from day to day with a negative mindset that keeps us trapped in a state of poor self-esteem, unable to see new possibilities for our future. This is a harsh reality that many of us face. As a result, it shouldn't come as a surprise that on a mental, emotional and spiritual note, more and more of us are battling depression, anxiety, loneliness and mood disorders, while physically we suffer from increased muscle tension, headaches, back and neck pain, digestive problems, sleep disorders, trouble concentrating, diabetes, heart disease, high cholesterol, high blood pressure, and some forms of cancer. I'm not saying that these conditions are all due to stress and negative mindset. It is, however, my belief that stress and negative mindset are strong contributing factors to many of these health problems. I also believe that stress and negative mindset are major contributors to the food and weight issues that so many of us face. What I'm suggesting is that there is a clear link between stress management, mindset, food and weight issues, and certain weight-related health problems. Poor stress management and negative mindset lead to poor eating habits, which can lead to being overweight or obese, causing increased risk for a variety of musculoskeletal problems and medical conditions. This is part of the ripple effect.

How we cope with the stress and pressures of daily life has a huge influence on our mindset, and how we eat and take care of ourselves. This is where the ripple effect begins. Here is a possible scenario. Does any of this sound familiar?

- *You wake up not feeling particularly refreshed or excited about the day ahead.*

- *You're feeling overtired, so you drink caffeinated coffee or maybe your favourite caffeinated soft drinks throughout the day to stay awake.*

- *You either have a small breakfast or skip breakfast completely, and end up eating some sort of fast food or restaurant food for lunch because you didn't feel like making lunch the night before.*

- *You finish lunch and now feel bloated and uncomfortable.*

- *You were probably so hungry by lunch time that you overate, and it probably wasn't a great meal choice, with either too much salt, fat, sugar or calories, and very little fibre.*

- *So now you take some antacids to relieve the bloating, heartburn, gas or acid reflux.*

- *Later in the afternoon, you have trouble concentrating, and start to get a headache from either trying to manage your work load or from sheer boredom. For quick relief, you take a couple of aspirin or other headache medication.*

- *At about 3:00 p.m., the sugar and starch cravings hit hard, so you can't help but reach for some chocolate, cookies, cake, chips or your other favourite sweet or starchy treats to satisfy the craving and calm you down.*

- *It's the late afternoon and you've been sitting at the computer for hours on end. You notice that your back and neck are starting to get sore from all of the sitting and muscle tension.*

- *Then your boss says or does something to reinforce your feeling that you are under-valued and under-appreciated in the workplace. You feel tightness in your chest or your jaw clenches in response, as you repress your true feelings of anger and frustration. You wish you had some food to eat, or maybe a nice glass of wine or beer, to calm you down and make you feel better.*

- *It's finally time to go home and you sit in traffic for over 30 minutes. Wanting to just get home, you're now furious with the other drivers driving the speed limit in the fast lane.*

- *You finally get home where your partner rants about his/her bad day and the kids are misbehaving. Nobody feels like planning and preparing a meal, so you order the family's favourite all-dressed, thick crust pizza because it's fast, easy and convenient.*

- *You have a couple glasses of wine or other alcoholic beverage to unwind from the day, get dinner over with, and help the kids with their homework. By this time, you're so tired that you can't wait to plop down in front of the television with your favourite snack food close at hand for comfort like a good friend, such as a big bag of potato chips, chocolate, cookies, or maybe a nice big bowl of ice cream. You had a hard day, so you tell yourself that surely you deserve to relax and have your favourite treats. After all, it's your reward for surviving yet another day in the rat race.*

- *Eventually you go to bed feeling depressed and anxious about your appearance, and/or your health, and/or the difficulties at work, and/or your relationship, and/or the problems your little one is having in school. Perhaps you take an anti-depressant or sleep medication to help stop the persistent mind chatter and fall asleep.*

- *After a fitful sleep, you wake up and do it all over again.*

This is one example of the ripple effects of being overtired, over-stressed and unsatisfied in life. Food and alcohol can become a way of self-medicating to relieve yourself of the mental and emotional aspects of that which makes you human. It helps to numb you so that you can go on behaving like a machine that doesn't think or feel.

Obsession with Youth, Sex and Beauty

It's not difficult to see what our society values as important and worthy. Everywhere you look, there are billboards and advertisements filled with beautiful, young men and women with perfect hair, eyes and teeth, and slim, attractive figures. We are obsessed with our outward appearance, striving for an ideal of youth, sexiness and beauty. Sadly, we are so influenced by what we see in the media that, as a result, many of us who do not fit the ideal image, end up feeling less worthy as people. Although men are also becoming more and more affected by these images, women have been vulnerable to this phenomenon for decades, if not centuries.

We tend to constantly berate ourselves for how we look, always searching for ways to improve by either losing weight, getting in better shape, changing our hair style or colour, or buying new clothes, cosmetics, shoes, jewelry, perfume, and fashion accessories. It's as if we can never quite feel *"good enough"*. Not all of us fall into this category, but too many do. When we don't feel that we look good on the outside, we often don't feel good about ourselves on the inside. We tend to judge our own self-worth as a person based on our outward appearance and the number we see on the scale. It's sad perhaps, but it's reality. As a result, many of us suffer from poor self-image, lowered self-esteem and an obsession with food and weight.

This food and weight obsession can lead to eating disorders, including anorexia, bulimia, and yo-yo dieting, where you drop weight quickly on a highly restrictive diet, and then gain it all back as soon as you go back to old eating habits. Perhaps yo-yo dieting is not classified as an eating disorder by most people, but given the long-term effects on health, metabolism and self-esteem, I definitely classify it as a type of eating disorder. Part of overcoming any eating disorder is learning how to reprogram your relationship with food and your inner-self. That's what this book is all about. However, this book does not replace psychotherapy. If you have serious issues from your past that you need to resolve, please seek the help of a trained professional.

We also need to think about what message all this yo-yo dieting is sending to our young children in the home. What are our children supposed to think about food, weight and body-image when mom or dad changes diets every week, and eats differently from the rest of the family, getting rid of carbohydrates one week, and then only eating grapefruit and cabbage the next? Learning how to achieve and maintain proper eating habits and a healthy weight WITHOUT dieting, by eating healthily and feeling good about yourself, will make you a much better role model for your children.

Let's face it, food tastes good and makes us feel better. Food is joy. Food fills the empty feeling we get when we're either physically hungry or emotionally malnourished. It brings comfort and temporary gratification when we're feeling down, or when we're feeling up. As a society, we nurture with food. We gain comfort from food. We bond over food. We celebrate with food and reward ourselves with food. The problems arise when we are not in control of how we use this powerful fuel and support system, without which we cannot survive. We may take it for granted. We may allow it to have power over us, rather than us be in control. This is when your relationship with food becomes unhealthy. It becomes one of both love and hate. You love the way the food tastes and how it makes you feel in the moment, yet you hate the power it has over you and how you feel afterwards, when you look in the mirror or step on the scale. The more powerless you feel in its presence, the more you hate it, yet you can't seem to regain healthy control over it. So how can you re-learn how to eat properly? How can you reprogram your relationship with food so that it no longer holds such power over you? What are other ways to cope with the stresses of daily life other than food, alcohol and medication? We'll answer all of these questions in the rest of the book.

How to Rise Above the Chaos

To start on the road to eating better, feeling better and living better, one must learn to rise above the chaos and stresses of daily life. This requires the following four things:

1) *Desire to change*
2) *Willingness to change*
3) *Readiness to change*
4) *Commitment to change*

Many people say that they want to change their lives. They talk about how they wish things were different, and focus on all the things they feel are missing and going wrong. They live according to how they think things are *"supposed"* to be, rather than how they really are. They say they're willing to change, but yet they do nothing about it. In order to change, you have to believe that change is possible, and be ready to do what it takes to make it happen.

How do you know when you're ready, you might ask? You'll know you're ready when it truly becomes your most important priority, and you can commit to doing your best in every circumstance, with an open mind and open heart to learn, make mistakes, get knocked down and get right back up again. If you're like me, you'll hit that point when enough is enough, usually brought on by some event that wakes you up and shakes you out of the fog you're living in. This event becomes your turning point, a launching pad into the future, taking you to where you want to go.

My turning point came the day I got on the scale and saw that I was heavier than I'd ever been in my life. My clothes were getting tighter, and I was feeling more and more self-conscious about my appearance. I wasn't comfortable in my own skin. I was thirty-nine years old at the time, and had lost my mother to cancer the year before. Approaching forty, and in the worst physical shape ever, I started to think about all the health risks associated with being overweight and inactive. I had already battled cancer, so what more needed to happen to kick me into action? I decided that enough was enough. It was time to take back control of my health and weight. It was time to take charge of my life. I wanted to get back to a healthy weight and more positive self-image by improving my eating habits, increasing my level of physical activity and, most importantly, changing my attitudes. However, I knew that restrictive dieting or going hungry was not the solution. I knew I wanted this to be long-term. Therefore, I had to find a system that I could comfortably manage for the rest of my life. That was when my healthy eating and positive living journey began.

What do you think your turning point will be?

_____

_____

_____

_____

What has to happen to kick YOU into action?

_____

_____

_____

_____

If you've already had a turning point, what was it?

_____

_____

_____

_____

The problem is that many of us are by nature resistant to change. This resistance may stem from:

1) *Fear of the unknown*
2) *Fear of failure*
3) *Fear of making mistakes*
4) *Self-doubt*
5) *Lack of faith that positive change is actually possible*
6) *An underlying fear of success that keeps us stuck*

If you're like most, you'll probably agree that it's much easier to stick to the status quo than stretch yourself beyond your self-limitations, and take the risks and actions necessary to get unstuck from your daily rut. In order to move your life to the next level, you will need to look change square in the eye and say something like, *"Change, I'm going to take you on regardless of my fears and self-doubt."* Did you know that even the most highly successful of people have feelings of fear, anxiety and self-doubt at times? What makes them successful is their ability to keep these emotions under control, rather than be controlled by them. Successful people are able to take action and keep moving forward despite these emotions. They do not let these emotions stand in the way of going after what they truly want to achieve in life. They learn to deal with their emotions productively, and put things into positive, healthy perspectives.

To reach and maintain a healthy weight and positive lifestyle successfully, these same principles of learning and change apply. Lots of change will be required to reprogram your relationship with food; from the way you think about it, to what you eat, why you eat, when you eat and how you eat. You may also need to completely transform your views of yourself, others and the world around you to ones that are more positive, healthy and accurate. If what I'm suggesting is making you feel uncomfortable or fearful, please know that it's perfectly all right to feel these emotions. As I said earlier, it is natural to feel some trepidation and self-doubt, perhaps combined with a fear of either failure or success.

What I encourage you to do is, regardless of your fears and self-doubt, let these feelings come, and then let them go again. They may surface from time to time along your healthy eating and lifestyle journey, but I ask that you just accept them, and keep moving forward regardless. I ask that you believe in yourself. Give yourself a chance, and enough time to see results, as even the smallest of successes can be extremely motivating and satisfying. I encourage you to give this lifelong approach your best shot, and simply trust the process. Go with it. Let it happen, and keep it going as best you can, even when you simply feel like throwing in the towel.

Remember, this is NOT a diet. This is NOT something you go on and off of only to gain all the weight back that you worked so hard to lose. My intent is to help you discover a new way of life. With time and perseverance, you will find your own way that works for you. This is not about anybody else. This is ALL about YOU. YOU are at the core of this change. However, there is another ripple effect at play. If you let them, those around you will influence your long-term success, either positively or negatively. How you allow others to influence you during your change process and in adjusting to the new you is also going to contribute to your ultimate success. And, vice versa, you can also have a positive or negative impact on others in terms of how you manage the change process and adjust to the new you. How you manage your relationships with others will be covered later in the book.

I am very excited to now present to you the 9 guiding principles for healthy eating and positive living that make up The "A" List. Each principle is just as important as the next, and I recommend that you not skip any. My suggestion is to read the book in the order that it is written. Each chapter builds on the chapter before it.

"A" Principle #1:
Ambition

In order to change, you first have to look at your level of ambition. What is your desire for success? For long-term, permanent change, your ambition, or desire for success, needs to be very high. This applies to your healthy eating and weight control goals, as well as any other life goals you set out to achieve. Here are some questions to reflect on.

How important is it to you to take charge of your health, weight, and quality of life?

    ❑ Very high

    ❑ Somewhat high

    ❑ Not high

If your answer is anything other than **very high**, I ask that you think about your reply.

What is more important to you right now than taking charge of your health, weight, and quality of life?

_____

_____

_____

_____

_____

What needs to happen so that taking charge of your health, weight, and quality of life is your top priority?

_____

_____

_____

_____

_____

What, starting this moment, will you do differently, so that taking charge of your health, weight, and quality of life is your top priority?

_____

_____

_____

_____

_____

What is your purpose in eating healthy, controlling your weight and improving your lifestyle?

_____

_____

_____

_____

_____

Why is this purpose important to you?

_____

_____

_____

_____

_____

How are you hoping your life will be different once you've achieved your purpose? Give examples.

_____

_____

_____

_____

_____

How hopeful are you that you can turn these hopes into reality?

    ❑ Very hopeful

    ❑ Somewhat hopeful

    ❑ Not very hopeful

If you answered anything other than ***very hopeful*** to this question, I ask that you think about your reply.

What has happened that makes you anything less than very hopeful *that you can turn these hopes into reality?*

_____

_____

_____

_____

_____

What needs to happen for you to feel more hopeful that you can turn your hopes and dreams into reality?

_____

_____

_____

_____

_____

What, starting this moment, will you do differently to increase your level of hope?

_____

_____

_____

_____

_____

_____

Assuming that eating healthy, controlling your weight and improving your lifestyle are very important goals for you, that you know your purpose and are brimming with lots of hope, then ask yourself the following:

How motivated and determined are you to do the work required to achieve your purpose and make your health, weight and lifestyle hopes, dreams and wishes come true?

    ❑ I am very motivated and determined

    ❑ I am somewhat motivated and determined

    ❑ I am not motivated and determined

If your answer is anything other than *I am very motivated and determined*, I ask that you think about your reply and answer the following:

What is happening that is preventing you from feeling fully motivated and determined?

_____

_____

_____

_____

_____

_____

What needs to happen to raise your levels of motivation and determination?

_____

_____

_____

_____

_____

What, starting this moment, will you do differently to raise your levels of motivation and determination?

_____

_____

_____

_____

_____

When you have a high level of ambition, it's not enough to have the desire, purpose, hope, motivation and determination for success. You also need to be highly committed. Your level of commitment will be the foundation for all of these other success factors. Your commitment is what will keep bringing you back on track when your hope or motivation starts to wane. The commitment to your purpose will be what drives your hopes, motivation and determination.

How committed are you to achieving long-term success for your health, weight and lifestyle goals?

❑ I am very committed to long-term success

❑ I am somewhat committed to long-term success

❑ I am not committed to long-term success

If you answered anything other than *I am very committed to long-term success*, then I want you to think about your reply and answer the following:

What is preventing you from feeling very committed to long-term success?

_____

_____

_____

_____

_____

_____

What needs to happen to raise your level of commitment?

_____

_____

_____

_____

_____

_____

What, starting this moment, will you do differently to raise your level of commitment?

_____

_____

_____

_____

_____

_____

If you don't believe that you can truly change your eating and lifestyle habits for life, then you will continue to self-sabotage all your best efforts in order to support this belief. I ask that you really think about the following question.

Do you believe that you can permanently change your eating and lifestyle habits?

❑ **Yes.** I fully believe in myself and my ability to permanently change my eating and lifestyle habits. I may not have been as successful as I wanted to be in the past, but that was then, and this is now. I'm ready for a fresh start and a renewed commitment. I'm ready to change my life.

❑ **Somewhat.** I somewhat believe that I can permanently change my eating and lifestyle habits. I haven't had the greatest success in the past, so I guess I'm a little unsure I can really do it. However, I'm willing to give this a shot.

❑ **No.** I don't believe that I can permanently change my eating and lifestyle habits. I've been this way for so long that I don't truly believe I can change.

Before going any further, I ask that you seriously take the time to reflect on how you answered this critical question.

If you answered *Yes. I fully believe in myself and my ability to permanently change my eating and lifestyle habits. I may not have been as successful as I wanted to be in the past, but that was then, and this is now. I'm ready for a fresh start and a renewed commitment. I'm ready to change my life,* then I congratulate you. I admire your confidence and enthusiasm, and wish you much success. You are off to a great start.

If you answered *Somewhat. I somewhat believe that I can permanently change my eating and lifestyle habits. I haven't had the greatest success in the past, so I guess I'm a little unsure I can really do it. However, I'm willing to give this a shot,* please know that I can fully understand your self-doubt. If you've tried to reach and maintain a healthy weight in the past without your desired level of success, then of course you're going to feel a certain level of self-doubt. However, I ask that you let go of all your past attempts. I ask that you pretend that this is your very first attempt at achieving a healthy weight. Start with a clean slate. Yesterday is history. Just because something you tried in the past didn't work out as well as you would have liked, does not mean that trying something new is going to turn out the same way today. Again, it comes down to your beliefs. If you go into this with a negative, fearful mindset, somewhat convinced that it's not going to work, then let me tell you that you will do whatever it takes to make sure it doesn't work, just to prove yourself right. You will find ways to sabotage your best efforts, I can almost promise you that. A little self-doubt or trepidation is understandable, but I ask that you fight your way through it. I ask that you feel the fear and keep going.

When you notice those self-sabotaging thoughts, behaviours and choices setting in, RECOGNIZE THEM, CONFRONT THEM, and CONQUER THEM. They can only get the better of you, if you allow them to. I ask that you not allow yourself to be controlled by your negative thoughts, beliefs and self-talk. Make every effort to turn your negative self-talk into one that is positive. Even if you don't fully believe your positive self-talk at first, keep at it. Pretend that you are someone who has a positive mindset. Think of someone you know whom you see as a positive, upbeat person. Imagine what their self-talk must be in order to maintain such a light-hearted and positive attitude toward themselves, others and the world around them. Be bold and even ask them what their self-talk sounds like in their mind that enables them to sustain such positivism. Adopt the same style of positive self-talk and make it your own. Over time, as you start to have small successes, you will start to gain self-confidence and eventually come to believe your own positive self-talk. When the negative thoughts come, challenge them immediately. Talk back to them like a rebellious teenager. Then replace them with the newer and healthier positive ones.

If you answered **No. *I don't believe that I can permanently change my eating and lifestyle habits. I've been this way for so long that I don't truly believe I can change,*** then you have a lot of work ahead of you. That may sound a bit disheartening, but it doesn't have to be. Remember, you've probably been a certain way most of your life. You didn't become who you are overnight. You've been programmed to believe certain things about yourself from your interpretation of your own experiences combined with the feedback you've had from your parents, teachers and others around you. When you start to confront and challenge your programming, and dismantle it one bite at a time, you will not only improve your eating, exercise and other lifestyle habits, but you will start to become the person you truly want to be, not just on the outside, but on the inside too. This will be a powerful journey for you. Your challenge will be to keep an open mind, be flexible, and be open to a future that you may never have previously dreamed possible.

Allow good things to happen. Enjoy your successes, and appreciate your hard work to overcome your challenges. Be graceful. Be forgiving of yourself. Seek help from an outside professional such as a weight management and lifestyle counselor, who can give you objective feedback and help you gain new and healthier perspectives. However, if you're suffering from serious depression, fatigue or acute anxiety, you may be best to first visit a medical doctor to rule out any medical or serious mental health conditions. Once these are eliminated, it's important to find out the background and area of expertise of the professional you are considering. It's also important that you feel safe, open and trusting with this person. You don't have to do this alone. Unless you start believing in yourself, and giving yourself a chance to prove that you can do this, you will not be able to achieve long-term success. You will continue to jump from one diet to the next, only to shed your unwanted pounds and put them all back on, and then some. You will not be able to end the cycle until you decide that you are ready, willing and able to commit yourself to creating positive and meaningful change for a healthier and happier life.

Sometimes there are conscious or unconscious reasons why you may want to secretly keep the weight on, or maybe even continue to gain weight. I ask that you give some serious thought to the next question.

What underlying reason might you have for keeping the weight on?

_____

_____

_____

_____

_____

_____

This last question may seem odd, as you might wonder what reason could there possibly be for keeping the weight on? I ask this question to my counseling clients and am no longer surprised by the answers. When asked if there might be a reason to keep the excess weight on, clients are often still for a few moments, without an immediate response. I remember the following answer, that has always stood out in my mind. See if anything in the following reply rings true for you.

The client told me that she was disgusted with her appearance and her lack of control over herself and her life. She was very unhappy inside, and blamed her unhappiness on her weight. In reflecting on this question, she realized that as much as she said she wanted to lose the weight, she was simultaneously afraid. Her fear was that once she lost the weight, she might still be unhappy and could no longer blame it on her weight. She admitted to herself that she used her weight as an excuse for her unhappiness. If she removed that excuse and still found herself to be unhappy, what then? Her fear was that she might actually have to confront her life and deal with the true sources of her unhappiness, but was not ready to do so.

This was an enormous revelation for her. It meant that she had a decision to make. Either she was ready to do what it took to change her life, or not. Changing your weight does mean changing your life. Yes, change may seem a bit scary. Yes, change does take commitment. Yes, change does mean reprogramming how you see yourself, others and the world around you. However, it is through change that you will not only shed your unwanted pounds and keep them off, but evolve as a whole person. You will not only see changes in your physical body, but also in the way you think, how you feel and how you live your life. You will recognize and seize new opportunities to learn and grow.

This is your chance to take a stand for yourself, so you can live a fuller, more satisfying life. We all feel some level of self-doubt, fear and anxiety when it comes to learning something new and changing our ways, but what separates the more successful from the less successful is persistence, resilience, determination, trust, and faith. By taking the necessary steps to take control of your health and weight, you will learn and develop as a whole person. Allow for it. Give yourself permission to create positive and meaningful change in your life. Accept it.

I understand that some of these questions may have been difficult to answer. They certainly forced you to reflect. Perhaps you even discovered something new about yourself. I ask that you read over your answers daily, and keep working at the areas you need to improve on or gain more clarity on. This will help you feel the driving force of ambition coursing through your veins as you begin your healthy eating and positive living journey. If you keep working at improving your level of ambition, you will see that your motivation, hope, determination, and sense of purpose will grow to where it needs to be for long-term success. In your calendar, I ask that you pick one day each month to answer these questions again from scratch. Start with a clean page, and write your answers as if it's the first time you're answering them. Continue doing this for the whole year. You'll be amazed to see how your answers can change from one month to the next, as your ambition grows.

Are you ready and committed to enjoying healthy eating and positive living for improved weight control and quality of life?

Take my FREE online Readiness Assessment at

www.roslynfranken.com

"A" Principle #2:
Attitude

I've learned through my own and others' struggles with food, weight, health and body-image, that certain attitudes open the door to long-term success, and others keep that door shut. Your attitudes are the driving force behind how you approach, feel and think about things. Your attitudes make up your outlook and your mindset in any given situation, and determine how you understand yourself, respond to difficult situations and solve problems. This does not only pertain to your weight issues. It pertains to every facet of your life, every goal you set for yourself, and every decision you face.

Where do your attitudes come from? Your attitudes come from your beliefs. We all have beliefs about things that, whether we are aware of them or not, influence every thought, decision and action we take. Our beliefs are the programs or codes that we live by. If you compare yourself to a computer, think of your beliefs as your operating system. We operate out of our conscious and unconscious programmed beliefs.

I can give you many examples of beliefs and attitudes that are counterproductive to healthy eating and positive living, but I want to highlight a few that were particularly difficult for me to work through and overcome, and are the most common with the people I have helped.

These specific attitudes are so important because by recognizing and overcoming them, it has not only helped me with my health and weight, but in every other aspect of my life as well. I suspect that many of you also struggle with these beliefs. By challenging the validity of your own self-defeating attitudes, you can learn to conquer them. Allow yourself to reprogram them with ones that are healthier and more positive. As a result, you will enjoy a much happier, healthier and satisfying life.

1) Perfectionism

"Perfectionism is self-abuse of the highest order"

- Anne Wilson Schaef

It's hard to say why I've always had a perfectionist attitude toward everything I do. Does it have to do with my upbringing? Perhaps. Is it simply part of my personality type? Perhaps. I don't believe it really matters WHY I've always been this way. I can't change the past, or why I turned out this way. The fact is I DO have this attitude, and unless I choose to change it, it will always be in control of me rather than me be in control of it. What matters is how this attitude has served me in my life and in my struggles with food, weight, health and life balance.

I believe that sometimes our greatest strengths can become our greatest weaknesses once they no longer serve us in a healthy and productive way. To some degree, I believe that my perfectionism was a strength when it served to motivate me to excel in achieving the goals I set for myself. However, striving to do your best does not mean you have to always be perfect. Therefore, it only became unhealthy in my case, when my need to be perfect was counterbalanced with a fear of failure. The unhealthy attitude of a perfectionist, means that when one achieves anything less than what is perceived to be perfect, one feels like a total failure.

The focus is totally on the negative, while the positive achievements are completely neglected or minimized. This creates an unhealthy spiral of self-destructive emotions that steals away the positive energy so needed to pick oneself up and get back on track. When it comes to healthy eating and weight control, trying to be perfect all the time is only going to stand in your way of getting to where you want to be. For your long-term success, you must learn to accept that you are human. Being human means not being perfect all the time. I, therefore, ask that you learn to let go of your unrealistic attitude of perfectionism and accept that you will never be perfect ALL of the time. Here are some questions to reflect on to help you overcome your perfectionist attitudes:

Do you feel a strong need to be perfect when trying to eat healthy, control your weight and improve your lifestyle? If yes, what typically happens? Give examples.

_____

_____

_____

_____

_____

How do you think this need for perfection has helped you when trying to eat healthy, control your weight and improve your lifestyle? Give examples.

_____

_____

_____

_____

_____

How do you think this need for perfection has hindered you when trying to eat healthy, control your weight and improve your lifestyle? Give examples.

_____

_____

_____

_____

_____

How do you feel when you achieve anything less than your ideal of perfection, when trying to eat healthy, control your weight and improve your lifestyle? Give examples.

_____

_____

_____

_____

_____

What do you do to cope when you feel this way? Give examples.

_____

_____

_____

_____

_____

How might your life be different if you could let go of your need to be perfect all the time in everything you apply yourself to, especially when trying to eat healthy, control your weight and improve your lifestyle?

_____

_____

_____

_____

_____

What needs to happen for you to let go of your perfectionist attitude, especially when trying to eat healthy, control your weight and improve your lifestyle?

_____

_____

_____

_____

_____

What, as of this moment, will you do differently to let go of your perfectionist attitude?

_____

_____

_____

_____

_____

Following, is a wonderful poem to help you understand the influence that the word *"Failure"* can have on your life.

Failure

*It's only a word
But it carries with it so much pain
and so little concern
so much frustration and so little respect,
so much stress and so little understanding
that people spend their lives
running through their days
in the hope of avoiding the long arm
of this little word.
To test our vision, you must risk failure.
To temper your ego,
you must attempt the impossible.
To tell your story,
you must take a chance.
To see beyond the horizon,
you must spread your wings.
To be all you can be,
you must stretch, flex, try,
and go beyond your proven limits.
To bridge the silence,
you must risk rejection.
To advance into the unknown,
you must risk the peril
of all your previous beliefs and emotions
that feel so secure.
Failure is not negative.
It is a teacher.
It molds, refines, and polishes you
so that one day
your light will shine for all to see.
It isn't the failure you experience
that will determine your destiny,
but your next step and then the next
that will tell the story of your life.*

-Tim Connor

2) People Pleaser

I have struggled with what I call the *"plague of the people pleasers"* for as long as I can remember. What can I say? It gives me great pleasure to see other people happy. If I can contribute in some way to another person's happiness, it makes me happy. There is nothing wrong with this up to a point. What I've learned, is that my need to please others becomes unhealthy and counterproductive, if and when I allow it to prevent me from getting my own needs met. Taking my *"people pleaser"* attitude to the extreme suggests that the other person's happiness is more important than my own. In terms of healthy eating and weight control, here are some examples of how this attitude can create inner conflict and potential food problems.

Many clients tell me that after-dinner eating habits are some of the most difficult to change, especially when others are involved. See if you can identify with this client's story.

Every night after dinner at about 9:00 p.m., she and her husband would either share a big bag of potato chips, or have a big bowl of ice cream while watching television. This was a ritual that they both enjoyed together. The problem was that every time it rolled around to 9:00 p.m., she would go upstairs on automatic pilot, and without thinking, prepare the treats and then eat them, simply because that was what they did together, and not because she really wanted or needed them. It was never questioned.

When I started working with her, and asked her how she thought this ritual was affecting her weight and self-esteem, she said that it made her feel powerless because she never felt like she had a choice. She was too afraid to change the routine because she was worried that her husband would give her a hard time about it. Although she enjoys chips and ice cream, she felt many times that she was eating it only because it was automatic and expected of her. Eating largely to please her husband, and share in this ritual, was not in her best interest when it came to her health, weight and self-image. Therefore, she had to learn to let go of her self-defeating attitude and start making gradual changes to turn this routine into one that was healthy and conducive to her long-term health, weight and positive living goals. This meant asserting herself more with her husband and explaining to him that, although she may start to make different food choices or sometimes choose to not have an evening treat, they could still enjoy each other's company. He would have to learn to adapt to her changes and give her the proper support she needed.

I once went to a friend's house for dinner where the host was serving lasagna. He served me what was three times the size of a healthy portion or what I would normally eat. He also poured everyone a new red wine that he wanted everyone to sample. The old *"people pleasing"* Roslyn, who struggled with her weight, would have accepted the plateful of lasagna and eaten every last bite in order to please the host. She also would have had at least one glass of the red wine whether she was really in the mood for it or not. The people pleaser inside me would have taken control.

I would have operated out of my *"old"* belief that leaving food on my plate, or not accepting the wine, would automatically mean that the host would feel offended. As a natural people pleaser, my automatic response would have been to do what I believed necessary to ensure the other person's happiness, even if it was at the sacrifice of my own best interests. Eating everything on my plate and drinking the wine I did not even care to drink, was not in my best interest. I knew I would not feel good about myself afterwards, but yet I would have done it regardless, just to keep the host happy. After all, his happiness was more important than mine, right? Keep reading and you'll see what the new and improved Roslyn did differently in this situation. But first I want you to answer the following questions.

Do you feel a strong need to please others when trying to eat healthy, control your weight and improve your lifestyle? What typically happens? Give examples.

_____

_____

_____

_____

_____

How do you think this need to please others has helped when trying to eat healthy, control your weight and improve your lifestyle? Give examples.

_____

_____

_____

_____

_____

How do you think this need to please others has hindered you when trying to eat healthy, control your weight and improve your lifestyle? Give examples.

_____

_____

_____

_____

_____

How do you feel when you do things to please others at your own expense, when trying to eat healthy, control your weight and improve your lifestyle? Give examples.

_____

_____

_____

_____

_____

What do you do to cope when you feel this way? Give examples.

_____

_____

_____

_____

_____

How do you think your life would be different if you could let go of your need to please others all the time?

_____

_____

_____

_____

What needs to happen for you to let go of your people pleasing attitude, especially when trying to eat healthy, control your weight and improve your lifestyle?

_____

_____

_____

_____

_____

What, starting this moment, will you do differently to let go of your people pleasing attitude?

_____

_____

_____

_____

_____

My New Attitude

As my healthy eating and positive living journey got me paying closer attention to food choices and portion sizes, I had to determine what was most important to me. Was it more imperative to please the host or myself? How worth it was it to go home feeling bloated and guilty from having made poor food choices, or overeaten terribly to please someone else? By challenging my automatic *"people pleasing"* attitude, I decided that pleasing myself and getting my own needs met was more important to me in this situation than the alternative. I changed my attitude to this — *if someone else is going to decide my portion size for me, then I do not have to worry or feel guilty about leaving food on my plate, or how the host may feel. How the host chooses to feel is not my responsibility in the first place.* I ask that you adopt this same attitude next time you are faced with a similar situation.

What the New and Improved Roslyn Did

In my example, with the oversized portion of lasagna, the new and improved Roslyn tried on her new attitude. As a result, instead of automatically accepting and eating it all like she would normally do, she chose to take control of the portion size. As the host was bringing the plateful of lasagna to the table, the new me spoke up and told him that I would not be able to finish such a large portion. I asked if he wouldn't mind putting two-thirds of it back, so as not to waste it. This way it would also not be on my plate to tempt me. I told him that if I was still hungry, I would not be shy to ask for more. Guess what? The world didn't come to an end. The evening wasn't ruined. The host did not run off to his bedroom crying because I didn't eat the huge portion he was serving me. We had a great evening and even got invited back. I never imagined being assertive enough to do something like this, but it actually felt very empowering.

Learning to assert yourself with others when it comes to social eating, is only going to help you reach and maintain your healthy weight and lifestyle goals. I encourage you to try it and see what happens. It takes practice like anything else. It may be uncomfortable at first like it was for me, but over time, your friends and family will get used to it, and learn to accept your new way of eating. They'll learn, for example, that you mean it when you say *"no"* to a second or third serving of dessert.

3) All-or-Nothing Attitude

The all-or-nothing attitude is closely linked with that of the perfectionist. By thinking in all-or-nothing terms, you set yourself up for failure. When it comes to controlling eating, managing weight and balancing your life, many people get stuck in this self-sabotaging attitude every time they fall off track. For example, imagine you're following a new diet plan where you can only eat certain foods, such as a low carbohydrate or no carbohydrate diet where you're trying not to eat any sugar, bread or other starches. It's Monday morning, and at 11:00 a.m. you eat something that is NOT on your diet such as a soft, chewy chocolate brownie. You just started your new diet plan, and already you feel like a failure. The sense of failure triggers the automatic guilt feelings and negative self-talk as you beat up on yourself for being *"bad"*. Yet, as the all-or-nothing thinker, at the very next opportunity, you will likely end up eating even more things that aren't on your diet. Your all-or-nothing attitude dictates that you're either going to stick to your diet perfectly all day long, or you won't even bother trying. You believe that since you already went off the diet or menu plan in the morning, you may as well write off the whole day and start again tomorrow. Only the next day, the very same thing may happen, and your proper eating, healthy weight management and positive living efforts are again in jeopardy.

Do you tend to think in all-or-nothing terms when trying to eat healthy, control your weight and improve your lifestyle? If yes, what typically happens? Give examples.

_____

_____

_____

_____

_____

How has this attitude helped you when trying to eat healthy, control your weight and improve your lifestyle? Give examples.

_____

_____

_____

_____

_____

How has this attitude hindered you when trying to eat healthy, control your weight and improve your lifestyle? Give examples.

_____

_____

_____

_____

_____

How do you feel when you adopt this attitude when trying to eat healthy, control your weight and improve your lifestyle? Give examples.

_____

_____

_____

_____

_____

What do you do to cope when you feel this way? Give examples.

_____

_____

_____

_____

_____

How do you think your life would be different if you could let go of your all-or-nothing attitude?

_____

_____

_____

_____

_____

How do you think your health, weight and lifestyle results would be different if you could let go of your all-or-nothing attitude?

_____

_____

_____

_____

_____

What needs to happen for you to let go of your all-or-nothing attitude, especially when it comes to eating healthy, controlling your weight and improving your lifestyle?

_____

_____

_____

_____

_____

What, starting this moment, will you do differently to let go of your all-or-nothing attitude?

_____

_____

_____

_____

4) Guilt, Shame and Self-Loathing

"Guilt is the very nerve of sorrow"

- Horace Bushnell

Typical weight reduction diets, programs and schemes are so rigid and restrictive, that the second you go off the prescribed plan, you feel like you've cheated, leaving you filled with guilt, shame and self-loathing. The very notion of cheating encourages these negative feelings, which only serve to further lower your self-esteem. As a result, you are at even greater risk to head straight for the fridge, cupboard or fast food restaurant in search of your favourite comfort foods to relieve the emotional pain. What I am asking of you is to eliminate the word *"cheating"* from your vocabulary. With my approach, there is no such thing as cheating because you're not on a rigid diet to begin with. I will teach you how to make conscious choices from a forgiving and appreciative mindset that will replace the negative notions of guilty cheating, shame and self-loathing. This was one of the most liberating steps in my own healthy lifestyle journey.

Do you tend toward attitudes of guilt, shame and self-loathing when you're trying to eat healthy, control your weight and improve your lifestyle? What typically happens? Give examples.

_____

_____

_____

_____

_____

How have these attitudes helped you in achieving and maintaining your health, weight and lifestyle goals? Give examples.

_____

_____

_____

_____

_____

How have these attitudes hindered you from achieving and maintaining your health, weight and lifestyle goals? Give examples.

_____

_____

_____

_____

_____

How do you feel when you act upon these attitudes when trying to eat healthy, control your weight and improve your lifestyle? Give examples.

_____

_____

_____

_____

_____

What do you do to cope when you feel this way? Give examples.

_____

_____

_____

_____

_____

How do you think your life in general would be different if you could let go of your attitudes of guilt, shame and self-loathing?

_____

_____

_____

_____

_____

How do you think your health, weight and lifestyle results would be different if you could let go of your attitudes of guilt, shame and self-loathing?

_____

_____

_____

_____

_____

What needs to happen for you to let go of these negative attitudes, especially when it comes to your health, weight and lifestyle goals?

_____

_____

_____

_____

_____

What, as of this moment, will you do differently to let go of these attitudes?

_____

_____

_____

_____

_____

5) Self-Reliance

Self-reliant means being independent and confident that you can rely upon yourself. My strong need for self-reliance came from my deep-rooted belief that asking for help is a sign of weakness, neediness and dependency. I feared that in asking another for help, it would automatically mean that I would be perceived as a bother, inconvenience or burden. I learned that part of my need for self-reliance stemmed from a desire to never feel that I was a burden or bother to someone else. As a result, I would rather rely on myself than ask for help. I'm not certain where this belief came from. Again, was it because of my upbringing? Was it just part of my personality? It is likely because of a combination of things that I can never be fully certain of. It doesn't really matter to me. The only thing that I can be certain of, is that it sometimes posed great obstacles to my health and happiness.

When I had my cancer at age twenty-nine, I learned a hard lesson about my own values and beliefs around self-reliance. One of the toughest things I had to learn was that it was okay to ask others for help. In my programming, I believed that it was important to always appear strong and independent and not to rely on others. I also did not believe that others would truly want to help me. I did not always believe or trust that others could help me in the ways that I needed most. Where did this leave me? It left me one day finding myself taking the city bus to and from a chemotherapy treatment, because I did not want to ask my then husband, or anyone else, to take time out of their day to drive me there and back. I was also under a lot of financial distress, and could not afford to take taxis. I would rather take the bus than ask for a ride. How sad was that?

It seems incomprehensible to me now that I allowed this, but the fact remains I did. Then one day, my cousin asked me how I was getting to and from my appointments. She assumed that my then husband was driving me. When I told her that I took the bus, she quickly offered to take me. It was hard for me to accept her offer as I didn't want to inconvenience her, but I had to start thinking differently if I wanted to take care of myself properly. What would it say about my self-worth and self-respect if I refused her offer? Was I not worth being driven to my chemotherapy treatments? When she said that she would love to take me and that there's no way I should be taking the bus, I had to accept that maybe she enjoyed knowing that she was helping me, the same way I enjoy the feeling I get from assisting others. This was a turning point for me. I learned that it was okay to let others be there for me and that it did not make me a weaker person. When she offered to help me, I immediately started to worry about things like *"What happens if she's late? What happens if she can't make it at the last moment?"* I had to learn to trust and just let things happen. I had to stop worrying about all the *"What ifs?"* In fact, I believe now that reaching out to others and asking for help when I need it, is actually a strength. I also believe that learning to trust others is important, as long as I accept that nobody is perfect.

The reason I am sharing this personal story with you, is because I believe that the attitude of self-reliance, and the need to always appear independent and strong, can have a detrimental impact on your ability to achieve and maintain the long-term health, weight and lifestyle results you so desire. Too many people feel that they should be able to do everything on their own, including eating healthy and controlling their weight, but, truth be told, it's perfectly okay to reach out for help and support. If you've been having trouble losing weight on your own, or getting the proper personal support you need, then give yourself a gift and reach out for the proper help. If over-burdened by your daily To-Do list, then learn to share the responsibilities with others, ask for help and learn not to over-promise to others or overextend yourself. Learn to trust others to get the job done, even if it's not exactly in the same way or time-frame that you would do it. You also need to be clear in communicating your expectations to others, and letting go if they fail to meet your standards of perfection. Reaching out for help, trusting others to help you, and letting go of perfectionism and unrealistic expectations of others, can be the biggest gifts that you give yourself.

In what ways is it hard for you to ask others for help and to trust others to help you? Give examples.

_____

_____

_____

_____

_____

How has this attitude helped you in achieving and maintaining your health, weight and lifestyle goals? Give examples.

_____

_____

_____

_____

_____

How has this attitude hindered you from achieving and maintaining your health, weight and lifestyle goals?

_____

_____

_____

_____

_____

How do you feel when you act upon this attitude when trying to eat healthy, control your weight and improve your lifestyle?

_____

_____

_____

_____

_____

What do you do to cope when you feel this way?

_____

_____

_____

_____

_____

How do you think your life would be different if you could let go of your need to always be self-reliant and start asking for help when you need or want it?

_____

_____

_____

_____

_____

How do you think your healthy eating, weight control and positive living results would be different if you could let go of your need to always be self-reliant and start asking for help when you need or want it?

_____

_____

_____

_____

_____

What needs to happen for you to let go of your need to always be self-reliant and start asking for help when you need or want it, to help you eat healthy, control your weight and improve your quality of life?

_____

_____

_____

_____

_____

If you were to ask for help, what kind of help would you ask for? What do you think you need help with?

_____

_____

What, as of this moment, will you do differently to let go of your need to always be self-reliant and start asking for help when you need or want it?

---

6) Must Always Be Liked and Admired

In struggling with my own food, weight and lifestyle issues, I learned a very valuable lesson the day I recognized my strong desire to always be liked and admired. I did not necessarily understand why this desire was so strong, and decided that, as of this moment, I would let go of my need to understand. I just accepted that this was a part of me that I needed to look at more closely. If you, too, have a strong desire to always be liked and admired by others, then I ask that you let go of wanting to understand where this desire came from and why it's so important. The way you are can be due to a variety of complex factors. I would rather that you put your energies toward looking at what the possible negative ramifications can be when this desire is held overly strongly, and what you can do to get it more in balance.

If you're like many, I suspect that what you believe to be true about this attitude is as follows: *"If I am well liked and admired by others, then I will be accepted and loved."* If this is true for you, then what would happen if someone did not like and admire you? You may believe that *"If I am not well liked and admired, then I will be rejected or abandoned and NOT loved."*

The problem with this attitude is that you may make choices in how you act and behave in different situations with different people that stem from a fear of not being accepted or loved, rather than doing what you truly WANT to do to honour your own needs, desires and wishes. This is closely tied in to the people pleaser attitude and also a desire to avoid conflict. For example, if you are in a relationship, you may presume that certain behaviours on your part will win over your partner's love and admiration because these are behaviours that you believe are required. If these behaviours are real, genuine, comfortable and true for you, and contribute well to your own health and well-being, then there may not be an issue. However, if you are doing things, or behaving in ways, just because you think that is what the other person wants you to do, then you can run into problems. This can put strain on you personally, as well as on the relationship itself. In time, it can lead to you having feelings of resentment toward the other person that will ultimately cause you unwanted stress in dealing with these difficult emotions.

When you do things or behave in ways that are not real, genuine, comfortable or true to who you really are, then you are living a lie. This may sound harsh, but it is the truth. You are simply keeping up appearances by repressing your own true self. You are not allowing your own spirit to come forth, shine and grow. Instead, you are stifling your own self to win over someone else's love, admiration and affection.

Here is my theory of how this attitude relates to negative food and eating behaviours. If you spend so much energy denying who you really are, then you are constantly in a place of deprivation. You are depriving your soul of being real and true. Therefore, when it comes to your relationship with food, you no longer have to "be" anybody but yourself. In your relationship with food, you might over-compensate for other areas of your life where you may constantly be depriving yourself. With food, you set yourself free. With food, you can be who you really are. Food has no expectations of you. Since you are not honouring your soul through your behaviour, you are instead feeding your soul with food. It doesn't ask you to be anybody other than you. Food accepts you and loves you unconditionally.

As long as I lived my life doing things and behaving in ways out of my fear of rejection and abandonment, I continued to struggle with food and weight issues. As soon as I started to honour who I really am, and really take notice of my own needs and wants, the weight started to come off more easily. Of all the attitudes listed here, I would say that this was one of the most critical. Here are the questions to ask yourself to help you sort through this attitude for yourself, just as I did:

How important is your desire to always be liked and admired by others?

_____

_____

_____

_____

_____

How has this attitude helped you in achieving and maintaining your health, weight and lifestyle goals? Give examples.

_____

_____

_____

_____

_____

How has this attitude hindered you from achieving and maintaining your your health, weight and lifestyle goals? Give examples.

_____

_____

_____

_____

_____

How do you feel when you make food and life choices out of your desire to always be liked and admired?

_____

_____

_____

_____

_____

What do you do to cope when you feel this way?

_____

_____

_____

_____

_____

How do you think your life would be different if you could let go of your desire to always be liked and admired by others?

_____

_____

_____

_____

_____

How do you think your proper health, weight and lifestyle results would be different if you could let go of your strong desire to always be liked and admired?

_____

_____

_____

_____

_____

What needs to happen for you to let go of your strong desire to always be liked and admired, especially when it comes to healthy eating, weight control and improving your lifestyle?

_____

_____

_____

_____

What, as of this moment, will you do differently to start letting go of your strong desire to always be liked and admired?

_____

_____

_____

_____

7) The Quick Fix

As previously discussed, our fast-paced, ever-changing society relies heavily on quick fixes and band-aid solutions. We don't want to have to wait for anything. We're impatient and easily frustrated when things don't happen as quickly as we'd like them to. Unfortunately, reality is such that when it comes to weight reduction, the quick fix attitude simply does not work. You already know that or you probably wouldn't be reading this book. However, it may still be a concept you have not yet fully accepted. I ask that you find a way to accept that gradual weight reduction is not only more effective long-term, it is also kinder to your body, mind and spirit. Here are the questions I had to reflect on in order to let go of my attachment to the quick fix attitude. Answer these for yourself and see what you can do to let it go.

Do you tend to always look for the quick fix solution when trying to eat healthy, control your weight and improve your quality of life? If yes, what typically happens? Give examples.

_____

_____

_____

_____

How has this quick fix attitude helped you when trying to eat healthy, control your weight and improve your quality of life? Give examples.

_____

_____

_____

_____

How has this quick fix attitude hindered you when trying to eat healthy, control your weight and improve your quality of life? Give examples.

_____

_____

_____

_____

_____

How do you feel when this quick fix attitude only yields you temporary results and you end up gaining back the weight you worked so hard to shed? Give examples.

_____

_____

_____

_____

_____

What do you do to cope when you feel this way? Give examples.

_____

_____

_____

_____

_____

How do you think your life would be different if you could let go of your quick fix attitude?

_____

_____

_____

_____

_____

How do you think your health, weight and lifestyle results would be different if you could let go of your quick fix attitude?

_____

_____

_____

_____

What needs to happen for you to let go of your quick fix attitude?

_____

_____

_____

_____

What, as of this moment, will you do differently to let go of your quick fix attitude?

_____

_____

_____

_____

Keep a copy of this poem with you as a reminder of letting go of the quick fix:

Patience

To wait with certainty - the art of allowing life to carry you.
Wait in the power of knowing what is possible...
Do not waver... Remain steady...
Remain true to your goals and allow life to carry you.
That which is worthwhile is sometimes created slowly.

- I -Ching Hexagram #32

8) *"I deserve it"* Attitude

Here's an attitude I bet you can relate to. This is one of the most popular attitudes I see in my clients. Imagine that you've had a really hard or stressful day at home or work. Nothing went as planned and you were met with one obstacle after another. You didn't get anywhere near as much accomplished as you intended to. On your way home, you start thinking about that apple pie (or some other treat you enjoy or crave) sitting on the counter. You imagine how good it will taste to eat it. You decide to have a small piece before dinner because you had a hard day and think to yourself, *"Damn it, I deserve it."* It's your delicious reward for surviving another day in the rat race. The amazing thing about this line of thinking is that it is totally illogical.

The most intelligent and rational people I know get trapped in this negative attitude. They put something unhealthy into their bodies as a reward for their suffering, or sometimes even to celebrate their successes. Yet all it does is lead to future suffering, since as soon as you've eaten it, you feel fat, you feel guilty, or it hits you when you get on the scale, see yourself in a photograph, or catch your reflection in the mirror. It provides momentary satisfaction, and long-lasting pain. Is the pleasure worth the pain? That is the question. Here are some questions to reflect on to help you sort through this counterproductive attitude in the same way I did.

Do you tend to reward yourself with your favourite less healthy treats when you feel you "deserve it" after a particularly good or bad day?

_____

_____

_____

_____

How has this "I deserve it" attitude helped you in achieving and maintaining your health, weight and lifestyle goals?

_____

_____

_____

_____

How has this "I deserve it" attitude hindered you from achieving and maintaining your health, weight and lifestyle goals?

_____

_____

_____

_____

_____

How do you feel when you give in to this "I deserve it" attitude, preventing you from achieving your long-term health, weight and lifestyle goals?

_____

_____

_____

_____

_____

What do you do to cope when you feel this way?

_____

_____

_____

_____

_____

How do you think your life would be different if you could let go of your "I deserve it" attitude?

_____

_____

_____

_____

_____

How do you think your your health, weight and lifestyle results would be different if you could let go of your "I deserve it" attitude?

_____

_____

_____

_____

_____

What needs to happen for you to let go of your "I deserve it" attitude, especially when it comes to healthy eating, controlling your weight, and improving your lifestyle?

_____

_____

_____

_____

_____

What, as of this moment, will you do differently to let go of your "I deserve it" attitude?

_____

_____

_____

_____

_____

What works for most is to turn your thinking inside out when it comes to the *"I deserve it"* attitude. As you're about to indulge in your favourite unhealthy treat, instead of allowing yourself to eat it all because you *"deserve it"*, change the self-talk running through your mind to *"I don't deserve it."* That is, *"I don't deserve to put this unhealthy food inside my body that will make me feel worse for it in the long-run. Instead, I deserve to be kind to my body. I deserve to be kind to myself."*

9) Forgiveness

"Forgiveness is the key to action and freedom"

\- Hannah Arendt

The most powerful change I made to my mindset, in trying to control my weight and change my life, was adopting an overriding positive attitude of forgiveness. It may sound simple, but it is actually quite profound. It is so easy to beat up on yourself every time you feel like you failed. It is so easy to let those negative feelings take over so that you just want to give up and quit trying. It is just too hard to always feel down on yourself. It clouds your whole outlook on life. As soon as I decided to forgive myself for my imperfections, poor choices and negative judgments, I started to see a dramatic change in my whole outlook on myself, others and the world around me. My efforts to eat healthy, control my weight, and improve my lifestyle became much easier, as I eliminated much of the stress that was self-inflicted to begin with. I want you to reflect on how difficult it is for you to forgive yourself when you are less than perfect. I ask that you simply give some thought to the following questions.

How do you think your life would be different if you could forgive yourself when you're not measuring up to your ideal of perfection?

_____

_____

_____

_____

_____

How do you think learning to accept and let go of poor food choices and behaviours would enhance your health, weight and lifestyle results?

_____

_____

_____

_____

_____

What, as of this moment, will you do differently to forgive yourself when you make poor food choices?

_____

_____

_____

_____

_____

10)   Rescuer/Nurturer

Another key attitude I learned to conquer was my underlying belief that I must take care of everybody, fix everything and make everything better for those around me, always be the responsible one to take care of things, help solve everyone's problems and ensure that there is always harmony and happiness among all.

The problem this created for me was that I was so busy focusing on others, and taking care of others' needs, that I had no time or energy left to look after me. Being a strong nurturer by nature, I wanted to rescue the world. I just didn't realize that I was trying to do this at my own expense. I believed that taking time for me and my own needs and wants was somehow selfish. This was a hard lesson to learn. It may also be a hard concept for you to accept, as it is for many of my clients who suffer the consequences of this self-belief, when taken to extreme.

In my programming, the word *"selfish"* was bad. I operated out of the belief that it was not acceptable behaviour to be *"selfish"*. The image I had of myself was that I must always be a *"good"* person. My concept of *"selfish"* did not fit in with this image. I felt responsible for other people's happiness and well-being. To overcome this attitude, I had to reprogram my concept of the word *"selfish"*. I had to learn that I could not rescue others, and nor was it my responsibility to do so. I had to learn that there was nothing wrong or bad about taking care of ME.

One of my current clients, aged sixty-six, really grasped this concept. She put a big sticker on her binder that said *"It's all about me."* I thought this was priceless. She put it there as a daily reminder. She now puts herself first in that she gets in her daily walk regardless of other people's needs or influences. She has learned to not take on other people's problems as her own, and to not always feel responsible for their happiness.

She has learned that their happiness is their own responsibility and they need to own that, just as she was now doing for herself.

Do you tend to always want to rescue, nurture and take care of others?

_____

_____

_____

_____

How has this rescuer/nurturer attitude helped you when trying to eat healthy, control your weight and improve your lifestyle?

_____

_____

_____

_____

How has this rescuer/nurturer attitude hindered you when trying to eat healthy, control your weight and improve your lifestyle?

_____

_____

_____

_____

How do you feel when giving in to this rescuer/nurturer attitude prevents you from eating healthy, controlling your weight and improving your lifestyle?

_____

_____

_____

_____

_____

What do you do to cope when you feel this way?

_____

_____

_____

_____

_____

How do you think your life would be different if you could let go of your rescuer/nurturer attitude?

_____

_____

_____

_____

_____

How do you think your health, weight and lifestyle results would be different if you could let go of your rescuer/nurturer attitude?

_____

_____

_____

_____

_____

What needs to happen for you to let go of your rescuer/nurturer attitude, especially when trying to eat healthy, control your weight and improve your lifestyle?

_____

_____

_____

_____

_____

What, as of this moment, will you do differently to let go of your rescuer /nurturer attitude?

_____

_____

_____

_____

_____

All of the attitudes listed in this chapter are a recipe for what I like to call self-inflicted stress. If you can identify with any or all of these common stress-producing beliefs, then I ask you to challenge and conquer them. I am asking you to let them go, and try on something new.

"A" Principle #3: *Attainability*

One of the obstacles to successful, long-term health, weight and lifestyle results starts at the very beginning of the journey when you are setting your goals. Goals can give you a destination to reach, a final outcome to strive for, and a purpose to follow. Goals are what will drive you to keep motivated, focused and on track. However, if the goals are not realistic, you could be setting yourself up for failure and disappointment right from the start. Let's talk about goal setting for a moment. You may have heard that effective goals are those that are specific, attainable and measurable. These goals are usually accompanied by deadlines. However, from my own and others' experience, I've found that many of us will set unrealistic goals with unlikely deadlines, which create unattainable expectations. These impossible expectations, will more often than not, be met with incredible disappointment when the desired goals are not achieved within the set deadlines.

You can end up becoming so over-focused on achieving your future goals, that you fail to recognize and appreciate all the positive things and opportunities for learning that present themselves along the way. Therefore, it is absolutely critical that you set realistically attainable goals for yourself right from the start. In this chapter we will look at how to set realistic attainable goals and deadlines.

How I Used to Set Goals and Deadlines

I remember the countless times I would start off the New Year with a resolution to reach my target ideal weight of 120 lbs (because that's what I weighed in high school and when I last believed I looked good in a pair of jeans). I always decided that I was going to shed my excess weight by my birthday on May 13th. With each passing year that I didn't achieve my goal, I actually started the New Year with even more weight to shed to reach my target weight than the year before. How did I let this happen? In looking back, it's easy to see why this strategy never worked.

Each time I made my resolution, my belief that I could actually attain my 120 lbs goal weight was more diminished. If I didn't reach it the year before, and I was now even heavier than when I started, something was clearly not working. In looking back, I don't believe now that I was ever fully convinced then, that I could really do it. With each year that I failed to reach my goal, my confidence sank lower and lower. The last time I was about to fall into the same trap, I weighed 165 lbs, my heaviest weight to date, with 45 lbs to shed in 4.5 months to reach my target weight of 120 lbs by my birthday. That would mean a steady weight reduction of 2.5 lbs per week on average. For healthy sustainable weight reduction results, you should ideally shed no more than 2 lbs in a week. If I couldn't sustain a weekly 2.5 lbs weight reduction, then I'd have to shed even more than 2.5 lbs in some weeks if I wanted to reach my goal by my birthday. Seeing that I'd been making the same resolution for years with little success, I felt that maybe it was time to re-evaluate how realistic my resolution was to begin with. Did I really expect to reach my target weight by my birthday? Was I really prepared to do what it would take to reach my goal by my deadline regardless of the methods or challenges? Would it even be healthy? Would I be able to keep the weight off? When I stopped long enough to answer these questions, I started to see things from a new perspective.

1) Setting a Target Weight

As a thirty-nine year old woman, was it realistic, or for that matter, necessary for me to weigh what I weighed when I was sixteen in high school? Did I really need to weigh 120 lbs now to look better in a pair of jeans? I decided to drop the 120 lbs goal weight and just focus on getting to a healthy weight that I could sustain long-term through healthy eating, exercise and lifestyle habits. I decided that my new goal would be to get back to a healthy, comfortable weight that felt right for me at my age today, and that I could manage to keep to over the long-term. Redefining my goal immediately took off a load of pressure. Now let's look at how I set my target weight.

Instead of focusing on a target weight, I made my goals very small and manageable, so that with each success in achieving a small goal, I was that much more motivated to set an even higher goal. For example, instead of aiming to shed 45 lbs to reach my 120 lbs goal as I had always done in the past, I set out at first to shed just 5% of my body weight. My doctor had told me that just a 5% drop in body weight could minimize my weight-related health risks, including heart disease, diabetes, high blood pressure, high cholesterol, digestive problems, back problems and even some forms of cancer. As a cancer survivor already, and with a mother who died of cancer, and heart disease on my father's side of the family, I knew that health was the priority. My attitude was that if I focused on my health first and foremost, and learned to eat and live in a healthier, more positive and more active way, then the weight would eventually come off. As a result, I would reap all the other benefits such as feeling more confident in my appearance, and having an easier time shopping for clothes.

I weighed 165 lbs, so my initial goal was to drop 5% of my body weight, which was approximately 8 lbs, to take me to 157 lbs. It was a lot more realistic and manageable for me to think in terms of 8 lbs instead of 45 lbs. It felt attainable. I actually felt relieved of the pressure that the number 45 was putting on me. Once I reached 157 lbs, I re-assessed and decided I wanted to shed another 5%, which took me down to approximately 149 lbs. By this time I was feeling great, better than I ever would have expected. I stayed at that weight for a number of weeks, and eventually my weight went down again. I finally got down to 135 lbs and my body just settled in at that weight. I may go up or down a few pounds, but have pretty much stabilized at this weight. In order to drop more weight, I would have to work much harder at it, and quite frankly, I don't know that I want to. I am healthy and in good shape, and want to maintain a healthy life balance as well.

In the following exercise, I will ask that you calculate 5% of your body weight. This is the ONLY goal I want you to set for now. If you can reach that initial goal without going hungry or feeling deprived, then you have achieved enormous success. That will be a time to celebrate (without lots of unhealthy food and alcohol, of course). Once you achieve this goal, then you can re-assess and determine your next goal. You will simply repeat the same process of defining your goal by 5% of your new body weight. Here is an example to follow. This is how it would work for someone who currently weighs 190 lbs. Simply substitute your numbers for what is written here:

Body Weight

	Example	YOU
Current weight:	190 lbs	_____ lbs
5% of current weight	9.5 lbs (.05 x 190 = 9.5)	_____ lbs (.05 x my current weight)

In the example case, 5% is equal to 9.5 lbs. This may not sound like a lot, but if you weigh 190 lbs and could shed 9.5 lbs without feeling hungry, deprived or like you're on a diet, then this would be a huge accomplishment to be very proud of. Once your weight reached 180.5 lbs, you could then aim for another 5% goal and see how that goes. That would be equal to another 9 lbs, which would bring you down to 171.5 lbs. From there you would re-assess based on how you look and feel, and set another 5% goal and so on, until you have reached a healthy comfortable weight that you can sustain long-term.

Now you have a set of smaller goals to work towards that are manageable and much less overwhelming than one big goal that could seem unattainable.

2) Measuring Progress

Before losing my weight, I used to weigh myself almost daily. I became obsessed with the scale. I ask that you ONLY weigh yourself once a week at the same time of day wearing nothing but your birthday suit. Your weight fluctuates so much throughout the day, that weighing yourself daily, or at different times of day, can give you a distorted view of your true weight. This may de-motivate you and throw you off track. I also recommend investing in a good quality scale that measures both body weight and percentage body fat. Percentage body fat is another important measure of health, aside from body weight. When you shed weight, you lose both fat and muscle. When you gain back the excess weight you shed, you don't gain back the lost muscle, thereby increasing your fat to muscle ratio. This is why it is so important to exercise and build muscle while changing your eating habits. We will discuss this in greater detail in Principle #5: Activity. In the meantime, here are some numbers to think about. If you go get yourself a good scale that measures percentage body fat, see which category you fall into according to the body range charts on the next page.

Body Fat Ranges for Standard Adult Women
(according to Tanita, The Body Fat Experts)

AGE	UNDERFAT	HEALTHY	OVERFAT	OBESE
20 – 39	Less than 21%	21 – 33%	33 – 39%	Greater than 39%
40 – 59	Less than 23%	23 – 35%	35 – 40%	Greater than 40%
60 – 79	Less than 24%	24 – 36%	36 – 42%	Greater than 42%

Body Fat Ranges for Standard Adult Men
(according to Tanita, The Body Fat Experts)

AGE	UNDERFAT	HEALTHY	OVERFAT	OBESE
20 – 39	Less than 8%	8 – 19%	19 – 25%	Greater than 25%
40 – 59	Less than 11%	11 – 22%	22 – 27%	Greater than 27%
60 – 79	Less than 13%	13 – 25%	25 – 30%	Greater than 30%

Another great way to measure progress is without using a scale at all. Instead, you could pull out an old pair of jeans, or some other snug outfit that you no longer fit into. Once a week, try on the article of clothing and see if it is fitting looser. You may also want to measure your waist, hips, legs, bust and arms, and keep track of your measurements. If your weight isn't going down as fast as you'd like it to, but you're losing inches, then you will still be able to notice your progress. Your clothes in general will also start to fit differently. Since muscle weighs more than fat, if you are building muscle through increased exercise, then you may melt inches as you're toning, but not necessarily drop as much weight on the scale.

On page 178, I've included a sample form you can use to track your progress on a weekly basis. Record your start date. Then enter your starting weight, current percentage body fat (if you have a scale that provides this measurement) and identify the article of clothing you are going to use as a gauge. You may want to use a belt as well, and count which notch you are closing it on. This way, you are no longer focused only on the number on the scale. You will also measure your success by your percentage body fat, and how you feel in your snug article of clothing or how your belt fits. Therefore, you have three chances to win success each week. Either your weight will go down, your percentage body fat will drop, or your clothes will start to feel more comfortable and looser, or any combination thereof. Any one of these three is a success, and all three is the absolute ideal.

I ask that you measure your results no more than once a week. I also recommend that you weigh and measure yourself at the same time of day, since results will vary throughout the day.

3) Setting Realistic Deadlines

As mentioned in the beginning of this book, we live in a society where we want everything quick and easy. We're all looking for the quick fix, band-aid solution, magic pill and the magic solution. As such, when it comes to reaching our desired weight, we often have a fixed date that we want to shed the weight by and that is TODAY. We want to lose it fast, and we want to lose it NOW. Well, I'm going to tell you that with that attitude you are much more likely to get discouraged, and go back to your old eating habits just as quickly as the weight may initially come off.

I asked myself, *"Why was it so important for me to have a rigid deadline?"* All it did was put immense pressure on me. Every time my birthday came and went, and I had not reached my goal, I felt like an even bigger failure. I could only focus on the weight that I DID NOT LOSE, without acknowledging or celebrating, for that matter, all the weight that I did manage to shed. And so once again I'd throw in the towel, go back to my old eating habits, and put back on the weight I'd taken off and more. To stop this crazy cycle, I decided this time to throw away the deadline, as I was not about to work hard only to give in yet one more time. I decided that if in any given week I managed to shed any weight at all, it was a success, whether it was a half pound one week, or two the next. As long as I was working hard at it with my health as the priority, even the smallest results would make me happy.

I simply eliminated the need for a deadline. So what if it took me longer to shed my excess weight? As long as I was reducing it in a healthy way that I could live with for the rest of my life, why should I put that pressure on myself?

I am going to ask that you redefine your goal of when you want to reduce your weight by. To start, I suggest you forget about setting hard and fast deadlines, unless there is a pressing medical reason to shed your excess weight, such as an upcoming surgery that requires a certain amount of weight reduction for safety reasons.

This is what worked for me, and I want you to see how this could work for you:

You already set your initial goal in the previous exercise. In the example I gave, this person's initial goal was to shed 5% of her body weight, equivalent to 9.5 lbs, given her current weight of 190 lbs. A gradual healthy rate of weight reduction is anywhere from ½ to 2 lbs a week on average. Therefore, in our example, to shed the 9.5 lbs, this person can expect to reach her initial goal within a range of approximately 5 - 19 weeks. The slower she takes it, the easier it will be to make her change in habits permanent, as it will be gradual over a longer period of time. If she pushes herself to shed 2 or more pounds each week, the changes may be too drastic and difficult that she will not be able to sustain them long-term. Why must it be so important to reduce your weight quickly? I ask that you answer the following questions and contemplate what your answers mean to you.

Do you believe you MUST set a deadline by which you MUST reach your final healthy weight goal regardless of the method and long-term impact on health?

❑ Yes

❑ No

*If **Yes**, is this belief really true?*

❑ Yes

❑ No

How has this belief helped you in the past?

_____

_____

_____

_____

_____

_____

How has this belief hindered you in the past?

_____

_____

_____

_____

_____

What do you think will happen if you DO NOT set a hard and fast deadline by which you will reach your final healthy weight goal?

_____

_____

_____

_____

_____

What do you have to change in your attitude to let go of any fears of not having a hard and fast deadline?

_____

_____

_____

_____

_____

What, as of this moment, will you do differently to let go of your need for a hard and fast deadline?

_____

_____

_____

_____

_____

If you do not set a hard and fast deadline by which you MUST reach your final healthy weight goal, the worst thing that can happen is it may take you a little longer to shed the weight than you'd like. However, it will be a lot less pressure and risk of shedding it too quickly or unhealthily. For example, imagine you're going to your best friend's wedding three months from today. You have this gorgeous dress hanging in your closet that you want to wear, only it is three sizes smaller than your current size. You decide it's no problem, you will just drop 30 lbs in three months to fit into the dress. A month goes by and you barely shed 6 lbs. 24 lbs to go, and the clock is ticking. The next month goes by and you drop another 8 lbs. Still another 10 lbs to go to fit into that dress. It's getting harder and harder to shed the weight. As a result, you find yourself going hungry and depriving yourself of all your favourite unhealthy treats, knowing that you have to do this temporarily to wear that dress.

By the time the wedding comes around, you fit into the dress, but you don't even enjoy the wedding because you have little energy from starving yourself, and end up gorging on the meal at the wedding and feeling sick to your stomach all night long. Was it worth it? And then what? The wedding comes and goes, you go back to your old eating habits, and in no time you put all the weight back on and then some. I am asking you to think about this seriously. If you are ever in a similar situation to this example, PLEASE go out and buy yourself a new dress that fits you today. If you happen to shed some weight healthily in those three months, you can always have the dress altered. Or work at shedding the weight slowly and steadily and when you get closer to the wedding date, then go out and buy yourself a new dress. This is a much healthier and less stressful approach, don't you think?

"A" Principle #4:
Awareness

*"We are what we repeatedly do.
Excellence, therefore, is not an act, but a habit."*

– Aristotle

I like to refer to this quote by Aristotle because it encompasses everything that is required to create positive change in any area of your life in order to eat better, feel better and live better. If what you are repeatedly doing is not aligned with who you are, who you truly want to be, and the life you truly want to live, then it stands to reason that you need to make some changes in what you are repeatedly doing. For most of us, this can be very daunting, as we are often completely unaware of the repeated actions that hold us back from living a healthier and happier life. Or, if we are aware, we are either afraid to change it, or simply don't know how to change it. The purpose of this chapter is, therefore, to help you become more self-aware and food-aware, so that you can understand yourself better, and learn how to make conscious versus automatic food and lifestyle choices.

What you repeatedly do is what I will refer to as your *"automatic habits"*. These habits are automatic in that you don't think about them, you just do them. When it comes to food, for example, your automatic food habit may be to reach for a bag of chips while watching your favourite show on television. You start eating the chips and next thing you know, you've eaten the whole bag. This is what I will refer to as *"mindless"* eating in that you were eating without thinking about what you were doing. If you stop and think about this for a moment, you can quickly understand that unless you become aware of your habits, you can't begin to change them. If you continue to eat and live your life in this constant state of mindlessness and unawareness, you will remain stuck in a rut, unable to move yourself towards greater health, happiness and satisfaction. In order to change, grow and move forward, you absolutely must choose to wake up. The first step to changing your automatic habits begins when you awaken to what you are doing in the present moment at the time that you are doing it.

Time To Wake Up

Typically, when you're dieting, you end up *"cheating"* or feeling *"guilty"* the second you eat something that you know was not on your prescribed *"diet"*. You beat up on yourself because you feel you've done something *"wrong"* and end up feeling like a big *"failure"* once again. You end up feeling negative, and depressed and perhaps like quitting because *"what's the use anyways"*, you tell yourself. Cheating, guilt, wrong and failure are all negative words that reinforce your self-sabotaging thoughts, feelings and behaviours. This can be very damaging to your self-esteem, and hence, your motivation and ability to achieve and maintain your health, weight and lifestyle goals. What if you could eliminate these negative words, feelings and behaviours from your vocabulary? The good news is you can, but it requires time, effort and commitment to change. It requires you to wake up.

So far, we've discussed automatic habits in terms of what you repeatedly do. However, what you repeatedly do starts with what you repeatedly think. Therefore, in order to change what you repeatedly do, you need to go to the source, and look at what you repeatedly think. What you think stems from your attitudes, beliefs and automatic programs from which you operate in the world. We already looked at some of the typical attitudes that keep people from achieving long-lasting health, weight and lifestyle results.

What you believe is the driving force for ALL that you do. Your beliefs are VERY powerful. You may not even know when they are at work, but trust me when I say that they are ALWAYS at work. Your beliefs form how you see yourself, others and the world around you. Your beliefs will determine how you respond to what is going on inside you and all around you at any given moment. Your beliefs have EVERYTHING to do with every food choice and life choice that you make. Therefore, you need to wake up and take notice of your beliefs around food and your relationship with food before you can decide what kind of changes in your eating habits you need to make. Here's an exercise I want you to complete which will help to clarify the point I'm trying to make here:

Which of the following statements are TRUE for you? Please check ALL that apply:

❑ I love sweets and can't stop eating them once I start.

❑ I'm addicted to anything with salt.

❑ I skip meals regularly.

❑ I can't leave food on my plate.

❑ I can't say no to food.

❑ I over-indulge to avoid feeling deprived.

❑ I eat until I'm overfull and uncomfortable, and then sometimes even more.

❑ I never know when to stop.

❑ I am controlled by my daily To-Do lists.

❑ I can't slow down my busy life.

❑ I use food as reward and comfort when I'm feeling angry, stressed, anxious, tired, bored, lonely or sad.

❑ I keep sweets and junk food in the house for the people living with me.

❑ I prepare meals according to the likes and tastes of the people I live with.

❑ At buffets I have to eat at least two platefuls.

❑ I eat more in social situations.

❑ I eat more when I'm alone.

❑ I never use a shopping list.

❑ I have no time to cook or plan meals. Most of my meals are restaurant, take out, convenient, ready-made, packaged, frozen, or microwavable.

❑ I always eat bread with my meal.

❑ I should be able to control my eating and manage my weight on my own.

❑ I make most of my food choices on impulse.

❑ I am ashamed of my weight and appearance.

❑ I drink alcohol regularly.

❑ I always sample, snack and nibble while I cook.

❑ I believe that eating right before I go to bed helps me sleep better.

❑ I view my self-worth as a person according to my body weight and the size of my clothes.

Now look at the language that is used in these statements. This is the kind of language you hear inside your mind, the words, or self-talk, driven by a powerful internal operating system that programs your every thought.

Each statement represents the story that you believe to be true about yourself and your relationship with food. You made up this story based on your past experiences or programmed patterns of behaviour. For whatever reason, you've been wired to define yourself and your food behaviours according to these types of statements, which influence your unhealthy relationship with food. The very language you use to describe yourself and your food behaviours has a lasting impact on how you will behave around food. For example, if you say to yourself *"I can't leave food on my plate"*, then as long as you believe that to be true, you will continue to take the necessary actions required to support that belief. That is, you will continue to always finish what's on your plate to prove to yourself that you are right about not being able to leave food on your plate. After all, who wants to prove themselves wrong? If you discontinued the behaviour, then the story you have on yourself as being *"unable to leave food on your plate"* would no longer hold true for you. Your story would then have to change.

When I went through this exercise with one of my clients, he told me, *"I can't say no to French fries."* This client's belief was that he was absolutely powerless in the presence of fries. Until he could start challenging the validity of this self-belief, he could not possibly change the belief or resulting behaviour. Therefore, once you become aware of your beliefs and habits, you then have to start questioning their legitimacy, and how well they are serving you. This client had to start asking himself whether or not it was really true that he absolutely had to eat ALL the fries on his plate. He also had to question how well this belief was serving him. His conclusion was that nobody was forcing him to eat ALL the fries ALL the time. Although he may have believed and felt that he had to eat all the fries, in reality he didn't have to. It was his CHOICE to do so.

When he thought about it, he also realized that this belief was not serving him well at all. It only got him into deeper trouble when it came to weight, health, self-esteem and overall sense of self. Every time he ate ALL the fries, he felt guilty and a failure. Yet, the next time there were fries in front of him, the cycle would be repeated; he'd eat the fries and then hate himself.

So how did this client manage to overcome his negative French fries beliefs and habits? How did he reprogram his relationship with fries so that he could take back control over them? Here's what happened. After slowly changing his French fries habits using the methods I will cover a little later on, I remember him telling me about the day he noticed he was confused. I asked him what caused the confusion. He told me that he was consciously eating fries less often, and decided on one particular day to pick a few fries off a friend's plate. He told me that he felt completely satisfied with just a small amount, and was able to say no after having just a few. Before this change, he would have kept eating them until they were all gone. He said he was confused because he thought that he *"can't say no to fries."*

I explained that because he consciously changed his behaviour, his story about himself was no longer true. He now had to come up with a new story to match the new French fries habit. I asked what his new story would be. He replied that his new story would now be, *"I can say no to French fries when I choose to. I don't need to eat them all and can be satisfied with just a few."* This was his turning point, when he realized he could do this for the rest of his life. He had permanently changed his relationship with French fries. He loved his new story and decided that he would stick to it.

Developing Your Conscious Awareness of Food and Your Food Behaviour

One of the keys to your long-term success for better health, weight control and improved quality of life, will lie in your ability to identify and overcome the unhealthy habits dictating your existing relationship with food. This means learning to simultaneously develop both your food-awareness and self-awareness. Without increased awareness, permanent change in habit is impossible. It takes practice to consistently maintain food-awareness and self-awareness, but, like anything else, it does get easier over time. In fact, it's been said that it takes about six months of consistent effort for new habits to become automatic. Therefore, don't give up, just keep it all going for at least six months, and you'll see how it will get easier and easier and more automatic.

Developing Your Awareness and Understanding of Food

In terms of increasing your awareness of food, you need to become conscious of what healthy choices are compared with less healthy choices. You need to re-learn what proper portion sizes of different foods actually look like, and how many of them you need to eat in a typical day. This way, no matter what food situation you are in, you can make effective choices in what you choose to eat, what you choose to avoid, and how much of your selected items to eat.

Learning to Make Healthy Choices vs. Less Healthy Choices

To achieve and maintain healthy eating, weight control and positive living results for long-term success, you need to learn to routinely pick more healthy options over less healthy choices as often as possible. This doesn't mean that you can never eat foods under the less healthy column in the following table. It just means consciously choosing the less healthy foods in more limited quantities on a more limited basis than the healthier ones.

The most important thing to remember is that if you make a mindful CHOICE to have something less healthy, then you cannot feel guilty afterwards. Once you make the switch from mindless to mindful choice to have it, then you also have to accept the consequences. If, for example, you're going to have a small portion of bacon with your breakfast on occasion, then have it and give yourself permission to enjoy it. Accept that on occasion you will have the bacon and it won't make or break your overall weight control efforts in the long-run. This eliminates the guilt. Just do it with a clear and conscious mind, as a well thought out decision, with consideration of the consequences, and then just let it be.

I suggest keeping a printed copy of the following table with you at all times for a quick reference until you have it memorized. Put a copy of it right up on your fridge where you can see it every time you reach for the fridge or freezer. Keep a second copy of it in your wallet, purse or pocket or even at your desk or office. If you often eat in your car, then keep a copy handy there too.

HEALTHY CHOICES	LESS HEALTHY CHOICES
Low in refined sugar, white flour, salt, unhealthy fat and calories. *High in fibre.* *Choose from these most of the time.*	*High in refined sugars, white flour, salt, unhealthy fat and calories.* *Low in fibre.* *Choose from these less often and in limited quantities.*

<table>
<tr>
<td>

- Leaner cuts of meat.
- **Chicken and turkey:** no skin.
- **Fish:** fresh, frozen or canned.
- **Fruits:** fresh, frozen or canned, unsweetened. If sweetened rinse under cold water to remove excess added sugar.
- **Vegetables:** Fresh, frozen or canned. If canned rinse under cold water to remove excess salt.
- Tofu.
- Quinoa (Keen-wa) – a grain high in protein.
- **Beans:** kidney beans, black beans, romano beans, chick peas, lima beans or lentils.
- High-fibre grains and starches including:
  - Whole wheat bread, bagels, English muffins, Tortilla wraps, pita bread.
  - Whole wheat pasta and couscous.
  - Brown rice.
  - High-fibre cold or hot cereals.
- **Soups:** home made, instant or canned, low in salt and not creamy.
- **Fat-free dressings and condiments:** mustard, ketchup and barbecue sauce.
- **Healthy fats:** lean protein, olive oil, avocados, nuts and salmon in limited portion sizes on a limited basis.
- Low-sugar and low-salt foods and beverages.
- Unprocessed foods.
- **Low-fat dairy products:** milk, yogurt, cottage cheese, quark cheese, cream cheese, sour cream, hard cheese.

</td>
<td>

- Fatty cuts of meat.
- Smoked meats, hotdogs, sausages, bacon, bologna, ham, and most fatty luncheon meats that are also high in salt.
- **Fast food:** burgers, fries and pizza.
- Refined grains including white flour, white bread, white rice and white pasta.
- Anything sweetened with white sugar, corn-syrup or artificial sugar: cakes, cookies, pastries, chocolate, soft drinks and more.
- Fried foods especially anything deep-fried: Be careful of Chinese food.
- Creamy salad dressings.
- Cream based soups.
- Regular mayonnaise, Miracle Whip and other fatty condiments.
- Unhealthy saturated fat: Butter, cheese, shortening, coconut oil and palm oil. Fat in meat and poultry skin.
- Alcohol.
- Foods containing lots of salt:
  - Boxed mixes for rice, potatoes or noodle dishes.
  - Most frozen dinners.
  - Regular canned soups and instant soups.
  - Most hard and soft cheeses and cheese spreads.
  - Salted chips, nuts, pretzels, cheese sticks, corn chips and other snack foods.
  - Most instant hot cereals.
  - Highly processed foods.
  - Prepared and packaged foods.

</td>
</tr>
</table>

About Healthy Choices vs. Less Healthy Choices

As you'll notice from the previous table, the healthy choices include items that are generally high in fibre, low in unhealthy fats, low in sugar, low in salt, NOT highly processed and lower in calories compared with the less healthy counterparts. It includes a variety of foods from all the major food groups including whole grains, lean protein, fruits and vegetables, healthy fats and low-fat dairy products. The less healthy choices on the list are typically the opposite. They are generally low in fibre, high in unhealthy fat, high in sugar, high in salt, and foods that are pre-packaged and highly processed. This LESS HEALTHY list DOES include what we typically think of when we refer to fast food, junk food, the usual sweets and desserts, or highly salted and processed foods. All you need to concentrate on is that the foods listed under the healthy choices simply offer greater health benefits.

Every time you make more choices from the healthy food list, and fewer from the less healthy food list, you are minimizing your dietary related health risks such as diabetes, heart disease, high cholesterol, high blood pressure and some forms of cancer, to name a few. When making less healthy food choices, as long as you give yourself permission to do so, and consciously choose your quantities, then by all means treat yourself once in a while. If it's not realistic for you to NOT eat these less healthy foods for the rest of your life, then, for long-term healthy weight control, you're much better off to fully enjoy them in limited quantities occasionally, than to deprive yourself completely, or eat them with guilt and shame. For example, if you love chocolate cake, then eat it guilt-free in carefully chosen quantities on a limited basis, and then let it go. You'll be much more likely not to over-indulge when you do have it, and find that your cravings for it lessen over time, thus making it easier and easier to resist temptation.

I often hear from clients that when they're on a *"diet"*, they believe that they can *"never"* have their favourite less healthy treats. The problem is then when they do have them, they vow to themselves that it will be the last time till they reach their target weight. They will completely deprive themselves of the treats, and then as a result, find themselves binging on them unexpectedly one day when their resolve is low. By binging, they over-compensate for all those times they denied themselves, filled with resentment for having to cut their favourite treats out of their regular diet to begin with. As soon as the binge is over, they come down so hard on themselves that it completely throws them off track and, for most, it is very difficult to get re-motivated and back on their *"diet"*. My attitude is that if, instead, you could just accept that you will allow yourself some chocolate cake or other treat in limited portions on a limited basis, then there's no need to over-indulge. You don't need to over-compensate because you know you'll eat some again in the not so distant future. This is much healthier and MUCH more realistic for long-term success.

I remember when I was a child and my mother would give me a less healthy treat, I would sometimes ask for more. Her answer was typically, *"No, sweetheart. You've had enough. Tomorrow is another day."* This was her way of saying that I could maybe have some more the next day, but for today I'd had enough. This is great when you're a child and your mother is there to regulate your portions, but as an adult, you need to learn to self-regulate in much the same way. Remember, tomorrow is another day.

Understanding the Less Healthy Choices

You'll notice that the foods listed under the *"Less Healthy Choices"* column are the problematic ones that we typically crave or have little control over once we start eating them. And, as you can see, they tend to be high in fat, sugar, salt and calories and low in fibre content. These are also the typical foods we turn to for comfort, instant gratification, out of habit, as a reward or treat after a particularly good or bad day, or when we're simply hungry, stressed or too tired in the given moment to care about what we're putting into our bodies.

When we over-indulge in these foods for any of these reasons, our self-worth is automatically diminished. That is, as we become increasingly overwhelmed by the pressures of daily life, we neglect doing what's in our best interest for our health, self-care, and happiness. It then becomes a matter of reconnecting with what is truly important and meaningful. If health does not bump its way up to the top of your priority list, then how can you expect to shed your unwanted pounds and keep them off? If it is only a priority some of the time, on a random basis, then as soon as you permit it to be deemed less important, you will be vulnerable to going back to old habits and putting weight back on.

Understanding Calories

A calorie is the term used to describe a unit of nutritional energy. Nutritional energy comes in three main forms including carbohydrates, protein and fat. All three are required in varying degrees to maintain optimal body and brain functions, as they each have their own roles to play. A healthy diet is one that has a good balance of carbohydrates, fat and protein, incorporating a variety of choices from all the major food groups including grains, fruit, vegetables, meat and meat substitutes, dairy and fat.

Your body requires a certain amount of nutritional energy (calories) to maintain a healthy body weight and proper body functions such as keeping your heart pumping efficiently, your brain thinking clearly and your lungs breathing properly. When you consume more calories than your body needs, the unused calories get stored as fat. This is why it's so important to maintain a good balance between calories consumed and calories used. If you routinely take in more calories than your body requires, and don't burn these extra calories through physical activity, then it stands to reason that you need to slowly cut back on your caloric intake and increase your physical activity.

However, rather than get caught up in counting every calorie you consume, which can get tiresome and is not always practical, I found it much easier to simply focus on making healthier choices more often and in larger quantities, and less healthy choices far less often and in smaller quantities. For example, if what you want or prefer to eat is high in fat, high in sugar, high in salt or high in calories, then it is something to be eaten in more limited quantities on a more limited basis. If it is low in fat, low in sugar, low in sodium and low in calories, then you'll want to fill up with more of these foods. Although salt doesn't necessarily add calories, too much salt is unhealthy and can lead to water retention, high blood pressure and other medical conditions. If you make gradual changes in how you eat in this way, and keep your health as your main focus and primary motivator, then the number of calories will automatically take care of themselves. I will talk more about proper portion sizes and recommended quantities a little bit later on.

It is much better to start by slowly cutting back on your calorie intake by 250 to 500 calories maximum a day and burning an additional 250

calories a day through increased physical activity. This may sound l
work, but it's not as difficult as it seems. When you start eatin
quantities of healthy choices more often than not (except for healthy fats
which must still be eaten in limited quantities) and are, at the same time,
slowly cutting back on the less healthy choices, your calorie count will
automatically be reduced. Also, as you simultaneously increase your levels
of physical activity, you will be burning more unused calories which will
help to control your weight.

Going to the Supermarket

Making healthier choices all starts with the foods you choose to bring
into your home. Therefore, knowing how to buy your groceries properly is
of utmost importance. To make healthy food choices at the supermarket,
you need to learn how to read product labels. If you're not the one who
typically does the groceries, then you need to either start sharing in this
responsibility or educate the person who is the primary shopper, so that
they learn how to make the healthier choices. The next section is designed
to give you the strategic information you require to evaluate the
nutritional value of your food choices and make smart choices. Go into
your food cupboards and pull out a few of your favourite products. Look
at the packaging and consider the following information.

How to Read Nutrition Labels

Learning how to decipher the information included on most food labels
will help you make healthier choices when going to the supermarket. It
will help you in comparing one product to the next to ensure you're
making the smartest choices possible. Here's how to read the ingredient
list and nutrition fact tables.

Interpreting the List of Ingredients

Most products include a listing of all ingredients on their packaging.
They are listed in descending order from the ingredient used most to the
ingredient used least. For example, if a label lists the ingredients as sugar,
flour and coconut oil, then you know the food item contains mostly sugar,
followed by flour and then coconut oil.

When you actually start to read the ingredients, you may not under-stand half of what is written. You therefore need to get familiarized with the following terms in relation to sugars, fats and salt.

SUGAR: If you see any of the following terms, know that these ALL represent some form of sugar. These include sugar, corn syrup, honey, molasses, dextrin and maltodextrin. Also notice anything listed that ends in *"ose"* such as dextrose, sucrose, fructose, maltose and lactose. These are all forms of sugar which should be eaten on a limited basis in carefully chosen quantities.

FAT: Fats can be listed as butter, margarine, shortening, lard, palm oil, coconut oil, hydrogenated vegetable oil, peanut oil or any other type of oil, monoglycerides or diglycerides.

SALT: Salt can be listed as salt, sodium, MSG, baking soda, baking powder or sodium bicarbonate.

Now look at one of the products you pulled from your cupboard. Take notice of the ingredients used the most.

What are the first three?

    1. _____

    2. _____

    3. _____

Is sugar, fat or salt one of the top three? _____

Is this a healthy choice or less healthy choice? To answer this let's go to the next step in reading the product label.

Interpreting the Nutrition Table

The nutrition facts are generally found in a table on the side or back of the package. Look at your product you pulled out from your cupboard and find the Nutrition Table.

It will look something like the following:

| Nutrition Facts | |
Per ½ cup serving	
Amount	% Daily Value
Calories 110	
Fat 0g	0%
Saturated 0g	
+ Trans 0g	0%
Cholesterol 0mg	0%
Sodium 135mg	6%
Potassium 80mg	2%
Carbohydrate 25g	8%
Fibre 1g	4%
Sugars 10g	
Starch 14g	
Protein 2g	
Vitamin A	0%
Vitamin C	2%
Calcium	0%
Iron	25%
Thiamin	45%
Niacin	6%
Vitamin B6	10%
Folate	8%
Pantothenate	6%
Magnesium	6%
Zinc	10%

It includes the number of calories and nutrient values per specified recommended serving size. Be sure to check the recommended serving size, since it can differ from product to product. This is important if you're comparing the calories and nutrient values of different products. You'll also want to look at the quantity you typically eat of that product, and see how your usual serving size compares with what is recommended. For example, if the suggested serving size of your favourite cereal is 1/2 cup and you're eating twice that amount, then you may want to consider cutting back your portion until you are eating a proper portion size.

The core nutrients found on product labels are typically fat, saturated and trans fat, cholesterol, sodium, total carbohydrate, dietary fibre, sugars, protein, vitamins A and C, calcium and iron, usually expressed in grams and milligrams. Some include more information such as found in the sample table provided. The % DAILY VALUES are typically based on a 2000 daily calorie diet. Your daily values may be higher or lower depending on your calorie needs, which vary with age, gender, and activity level.

Since men tend to start off with a higher muscle to fat ratio naturally, they can consume more calories than women (approximately 500 more calories per day for a total of 2500, depending on age and level and intensity of physical activity) and therefore, can eat greater quantities of fat, carbohydrates and protein in proportion to the greater number of calories. The more physically active you are and the more lean muscle you work at building, the more calories you may need to consume. Remember that muscle burns more calories than fat, so with a higher muscle to fat ratio, you will also be burning more calories. Your body needs calories to burn, so don't be afraid to give your body what it needs, especially if you are steadily increasing your level and intensity of physical activity.

Based on a 2000 calorie diet, the recommended daily intake is as follows:

	Quantity	Calories	% of total Calories
Total Fat	Less than 65g	Less than 600	Less than 30%
Saturated Fat	Less than 20g	Less than 200	Less than 10%
Cholesterol	Less than 300mg	-----	-----
Sodium	Less than 2400mg	-----	-----
Calcium	1000 - 1500mg	-----	-----
Total Carbohydrates	300g	1200	60%
Dietary Fibre	25g	100	5%
Protein	50g	200	10%

Calories per gram: Fat 9, Carbohydrate 4, Protein 4

FAT

- Notice that fat has more than twice the amount of calories compared with carbohydrates and protein. According to nutritional experts, no more than 10% of your daily caloric intake should be coming from less healthy saturated fats which, if you remember in the less healthy food listing, include such items as butter, cheese, cream, shortening, coconut oil and palm oil as well as fat found in fatty cuts of meat and poultry skin. Foods high in saturated fats include most baked goods such as cakes, cookies, pastries, croissants, scones, brownies, most muffins, granola bars, etc. Try to eat these types of fatty food items sparingly. We will talk more about managing fats a little bit later.

CHOLESTEROL

- Notice that cholesterol is not measured in calories. Regardless of your suggested caloric intake, experts recommend limiting your cholesterol intake to no more than 300mg in a day. This is especially important if you're over forty and a woman in your menopausal years, because as estrogen levels decrease, cholesterol levels may actually start to rise. With age, both sexes become more susceptible to high cholesterol and, therefore, have to start paying closer attention to the foods that they eat. Watching your cholesterol levels during these years can help improve your health as you grow older. Foods high in cholesterol to be eaten in limited quantities on a limited basis include animal products such as meat, butter, cream and eggs.

CALCIUM

- Notice that calcium is also not measured in calories. Regardless of your caloric intake, experts recommend feeding your body 1000 – 1500mg of calcium per day. This is especially important if you're a woman over forty and in your menopausal years, because as your estrogen levels decrease, your bones start to deplete themselves of calcium, thereby weakening their strength and increasing your risk of breakage in later post-menopausal years. Experts recommend that after age fifty women should increase their calcium intake to approximately 1500mg per day.

SODIUM

- Notice that sodium is not measured in calories. Regardless of your caloric intake, experts recommend limiting your sodium intake to less than 2400mg in a day. If you routinely eat items high in salt such as packaged rice, potato and noodle dishes, most frozen dinners, regular canned soups and instant soups, most hard and soft cheeses and cheese spreads, most chips, nuts, pretzels, cheese sticks, corn chips and other snack foods, most instant hot cereals and most other highly processed, prepared and pre-packaged foods, then start reading food labels and notice how high in salt they really are. For example, if you eat store-bought frozen lasagna, notice that the sodium might be close to 900mg per suggested single serving size. If you typically reach for a second helping, then you've just consumed 1800mg of sodium total in only one meal for 75% of your maximum daily requirement. Depending on how much salt is in your other foods, you can easily go over the daily recommended maximum. If you tend toward retaining water, or are at risk of developing high blood pressure, you may well consider limiting your sodium intake to far less than the 2400mg maximum. You can easily save a whopping 900mg just by having a big salad with the lasagna instead of reaching for that second helping. This will save you on a lot of fat and calories as well, so all in all, a highly recommended choice.

It's also important to note that as a woman ages into menopause, and as men approach their later years, sensitivity to salt may increase, leading to increased water retention, risk of high blood pressure and cardiovascular disease. Therefore, as you get older, even if you're not suffering from high blood pressure, you may still want to lower your sodium intake for increased health and healthy weight control. 2400mg per day is the maximum. Both men and women can minimize salt sensitivity health risks more efficiently by cutting it back slowly to 1500mg per day.

FIBRE

- Notice that it is recommended to eat 25g of fibre per 2000 calories a day. According to nutritional experts, most North Americans don't get anywhere near this amount because they're too busy filling up on foods from the less healthy listing. Aim for high-fibre foods, which have 4g of fibre or more per serving.

Start looking at the calories of some of your favourite sweets and fatty foods as listed on the nutritional labels, and you'll be surprised how even small quantities of high-fat, high-sugar items can pack on the calories. Read the list of ingredients.

Again, you don't have to sit and track each calorie you eat. However, I do recommend reading product labels and paying attention to the number of calories per serving as well as other nutritional content. If you typically eat two or three servings in one sitting, then multiply the calories per serving by how many servings you eat. Start eating smaller portions of your favourite high-sugar, high-fat, high-salt, high-calorie foods and you'll start to see a difference in your weight. For example, if you're used to eating six chocolate chip cookies at one sitting, and you start by cutting it back to four cookies, then you could easily save yourself a few hundred calories right there with only that one small change. If in that same day you would normally have a serving of French fries with your meal, challenge yourself to either leave a third of your usual portion of fries on the plate, or better yet, order a salad some of the time instead. This small change can save you another load of calories, easily. There, you've already saved yourself a few hundred calories without too much sacrifice. This way is a lot easier to adapt to, and more realistic to stick to long-term than trying to cut out your favourite foods completely. I ask that you don't feel guilty about having the four chocolate chip cookies or two-thirds of the fries on your plate.

Instead, learn to recognize your successes, and give yourself a pat on the back for not eating ALL six cookies or ALL the fries as you normally would. As long as you're doing something differently than you normally would in how you eat your favourite less healthy choices (assuming you're having less and not more), then you are going in the right direction. Eventually, you might want to replace the cookies with a piece of fruit or yogurt some of the time. This will save you an additional few hundred calories. Over time, you may find that you crave the cookies less often, and find yourself automatically reaching for the healthier choice. Believe it or not, you'll actually start to crave the healthier choices. So you see, it doesn't take that much. It requires small changes over time. Do that for a few weeks until it becomes easier and easier, and then slowly cut back again on your high-fat, high-sugar, high-salt, and high-calorie items.

It is MUCH better to make these types of changes slowly. If you cut back on calories too fast and too drastically, you will only hurt your metabolism in the long-run, making it harder and harder to lose the weight every time you try. Repeat this process till you are making healthy choices most of the time on a regular basis. I will come back to this topic a little later on with more detail on how to make healthier choices most of the time, and teach you how to make small changes that will yield big results.

I also suggest that you start a moderate exercise program to burn extra calories per day. Go for a walk. Take the stairs. Go for a swim. Do some weight lifting while watching television. Start VERY slowly if you're not used to exercising, to avoid injury. Every bit of extra physical activity counts.

Regular aerobic exercise is a great way to work fat and boost metabolism. Lifting weights is a great way to build muscle and burn more calories. Muscle burns more calories than fat, so more muscle means more calories burned. See the chapter on Principle #5: Activity, for further information on incorporating more physical activity into your daily routine.

About Carbohydrates

Carbohydrates are an essential part of a healthy balanced diet. Your brain needs carbohydrates to function properly, so I ask that you avoid those rapid weight loss diets that suggest eliminating ALL carbohydrates from your diet. The idea here is to learn what types of carbohydrates negatively impact your ability to control your weight and how to make small changes to yield big results.

Managing Blood Sugar Levels

Managing your blood sugar levels is important for healthy weight control results because when your blood sugar levels see sudden boosts, your body produces more insulin than is needed. The leftover insulin that doesn't get used up gets stored as fat. There are some carbohydrates that wreak more havoc on your blood sugar levels than others. We will refer to these as the less healthy carbohydrates. These include refined grains such as white bread, white rice, white pasta, white bagels, and white rolls. Other foods with lots of white flour and/or added refined sugar such as cookies, chocolate, soft drinks, pies, pastries, cakes and pretty much any type of commercial sweets are also big trouble makers. These are the types of less healthy sugars and carbohydrates that should be eaten in limited quantities on a limited basis because of their negative impact on the body.

Along with sudden spikes in your insulin, these foods actually trigger your brain to tell you that you're still hungry and want more, making them so addictive for some people. Doesn't that help to explain why it can be so hard to stop eating these foods once you start? To make matters worse, when you're overstressed and overtired, your body craves these types of sugars and carbohydrates even more because of the sudden energy burst they provide. The more stressed and overtired you are, the weaker your resistance to these tempting foods because of the immediate gratification and comfort they provide. The problem is that a feeling of fatigue usually follows the immediate energy burst. So what do you do to combat the fatigue? You go for more sugar and less healthy carbohydrates to regain your energy. It is a cruel cycle of nature, don't you think? It is one that will keep you spinning your wheels with your healthy eating, weight control and improved lifestyle efforts if you give in to your cravings and temptations each and every time. If you find yourself trapped in this unhealthy cycle, then recognize that it is time to implement some changes.

It's important to know that while your brain is making you hungry for more of the insulin-boosting carbohydrates, your liver is actually producing more fat. This is clearly a physiological response you want to stop dead in its tracks. Therefore, you have to make choices that don't trigger these signals to be released. This is even more critical if you're a woman over forty and in your menopausal years. Experts say that with decreases in estrogen levels comes an increased sensitivity to sugar and inability to process the excess insulin as effectively. More insulin is therefore released to do the same job as it did before, and with the excess insulin comes even greater fat storage, leading to the weight gain typically seen in women starting in menopausal years. And, just to add insult to injury, of course this excess fat tends to accumulate around the waist where it is also known to be most dangerous, putting you at greater risk of cardiovascular and other diseases. It is the fat found in the abdominal area that is highly sensitive to insulin. The fat cells in your abdomen tend to be the ones that are most sensitive to insulin and work the hardest at storing fat, which is why women typically see their waists expand starting in their early forties.

Men are not immune to the effects of this insulin sensitivity that comes as you age. Ever notice how as men approach middle-age they start to gain weight around the middle? For men it's often referred to as a *"beer belly"*, but really it is similar to a woman's expanded belly area that comes with age, hormonal changes and poor eating and lifestyle habits. Around the same age that women's estrogen levels are decreasing, men's levels of free testosterone are also starting to take a nosedive, while their estrogen and insulin levels are increasing.

Therefore, whether you're male or female, you want to manage your blood sugar levels as best possible, minimizing the amount of excess insulin produced so it doesn't get stored as fat. It is also important to note that while all of this is going on, your body is also unable to burn calories like it used to, so it's a double whammy. The less healthy, insulin-boosting carbohydrates can also be very high in calories, which will just be that much harder to burn. All the more incentive to change the way you eat by limiting the amounts of these foods you consume. You can still eat your less healthy carbohydrates from time to time, but the key is to consume them in carefully chosen quantities on a limited basis. You will also appreciate them that much more when you do have them. Or you will find that your tastes may change over time and you won't crave them as much. That is always the best-case scenario. You may find over time that as you eat fewer of them, on a more limited basis, they no longer satisfy you to the same degree that they did before.

Good News

The good news is that there are a few ways to better manage your blood sugar levels, so that you stop this out of control eating of insulin-boosting comfort foods. The first is to GRADUALLY increase your fibre intake, as fibre is another type of carbohydrate that has been shown to keep blood sugar levels more regulated, fill you up so you feel fuller longer and causes your liver to produce less fat. All in all, a pretty good recipe for greater health and weight control. Therefore, if you love the less healthy carbohydrates and sugars, then you need to find healthier high-fibre substitutes that will satisfy you and not leave you feeling hungry or deprived.

Small Changes You Can Make to Increase Your Fibre Intake

On average, we should be aiming to consume a minimum of 25g of fibre per day. Unfortunately, most of us do not eat nearly this amount. Since fibre is only found in plant-based foods such as fruits, vegetables and grains, this means that the average North American is not consuming enough of these fibre-rich foods.

If you're currently eating a lot of the less healthy carbohydrates, such as white bread, white pasta, white bagels, white rolls, and low-fibre crackers, then it's time to switch to brown bread, brown pasta, brown bagels, brown rolls, and higher fibre crackers. The problem with *"white"* is that most of the fibre has been removed, along with many important nutrients our bodies need. It is therefore recommended to choose *"brown"* over *"white"*, as often as possible. This is an easy switch to make that will make a big difference in your nutrition, health, weight control and improved lifestyle.

When making the switch, read product labels and look for the brands that give you the most bang for your buck when it comes to fibre. For example, if you're looking to stock up on crackers, read the labels. If your usual brand only has 1g of fibre per single serving size while another brand has 4g for the same serving size, then opt for the higher fibre brand. Also make sure to check that the grams of fat per serving are as low as possible. Less fat is always better than more fat, especially if it is an unhealthy kind such as butter, shortening, coconut oil or palm oil. Try to choose products with less than 3g of fat per serving and 4g of fibre or more. Fruits and vegetables have far fewer calories and less fat in general than most grain products, so if for example, you routinely eat too much bread and pasta, and not enough fruit and vegetables, then a healthy strategy to consume more fibre with fewer calories, would be to cut back a bit on the grain products, and eat more fruits and vegetables to fill the gap.

As for sugary sweets and baked goods, my suggestion is to slowly cut back on your portion sizes and the frequency of these hard-to-resist high-sugar, high-fat, and high-calorie foods. It may seem hard to believe, but the less sugar you eat, the less sugar you crave. I know that for you self-proclaimed donut lovers and chocoholics out there, this may seem nearly impossible. Don't forget that when you eat too much sugar, your brain will actually tell you that you're hungry for more, and you'll want to keep eating. You will crave more sugar. When you stop and think about the empty calories you're wasting on sugar, and the fact that it will make your brain make you hungry for more and be turned to fat very quickly, you have to stop and ask yourself if it is really worth it in the long-run. So next time you're tempted by your favourite dessert, try cutting back the portion slightly or, better yet, have some natural sugar instead such as a piece of fruit.

About Fat

Unfortunately, we've been programmed by the media in the last few decades to believe that ALL fat is bad. In seeking to reduce weight, most commercial diets and programs will tell you to stay away from ALL fat. What I suggest is learning how to incorporate both healthy and less healthy fats into your regular eating routine. To say to yourself that you will NEVER have any fats listed under the less healthy list such as cheese, bacon, chocolate, butter and cream, may not be realistic in the long-term. The less healthy fats are simply not great choices for your health, especially when eaten mindlessly and in too large portions on too frequent a basis. The bottom line is you will want to make healthy fat choices far more frequently than their less healthy counterparts.

For example, having an olive oil based salad dressing with your salad is far better for you than eating a salad with a creamy Caesar dressing. Therefore, when you're about to eat a salad, choose an olive oil based dressing most of the time and the creamy Caesar dressing on occasion as a way to treat yourself. In time, you may find that your tastes change and you won't even enjoy the fattier dressings nearly as much. Your body may actually start to crave the olive oil based dressing instead. As you age, your digestion and ability to metabolize fat may not be as efficient, which could cause health problems such as painful gallstones. Therefore, the sooner you gain some control over how much fat you consume, the less risk for health problems later on. For example, nuts and seeds are very nutritious, but generally very high in healthy fat and extremely dense in calories. Just because they are listed as a healthy choice, does not mean you can eat as many as you want. If you can fit them all on two fingers, then that is your desired portion size. They should also be eaten in proper balance with your other intake for that day.

Don't forget that foods that are fried or deep-fried are not only loaded with fat, they are also loaded with calories. Remember that each gram of fat has 9 calories, more than twice that of protein and carbohydrates, which only have 4 calories per gram.

About Protein

Protein is found in meat, poultry, fish, eggs, and dairy products, along with vegetables, beans, and other plant sources. Your body needs a certain amount of protein to maintain, repair and replace body tissue, among many other important bodily functions. The best sources of protein are lean cuts of meat, chicken or turkey with skin removed, tuna, salmon and other fish, eggs and low-fat dairy products such as milk, yogurt, cheese, cottage cheese, buttermilk and quark cheese as well as beans, especially when combined with a starch such as rice, pasta or couscous (see recipes at back of book).

IMPORTANT NOTE: *High protein/low carbohydrate diets have become increasingly popular in recent years. These types of diets can be dangerous to your* *health and are NOT recommended. For example, they can cause kidney problems because of how much harder the body must work to process all the excess proteins. A male friend of mine went on one of these types of diet and woke up one morning unable to urinate. He went to the doctor and discovered that his kidneys had shut down. He was advised to get off the high protein/ low carbohydrate diet immediately. His kidneys never fully recovered. Too much protein can also lead to high cholesterol and gout, and they can be high in fat, leading to an increased risk of heart disease.*

About Water

Drinking plenty of water is important in boosting your health, controlling your weight and maintaining good energy levels throughout the day. Your body needs water to help eliminate wastes, keep your body cool and, in terms of health and weight control, helps to metabolize fats and other foods. To reap all these wonderful rewards, it is recommended that you drink one cup (8 oz) of water for every 20 lbs of weight. Therefore, the more you weigh, the more water your body needs. If you are losing a lot of water through perspiration due to heat or physical activity, it is recommended that you drink even more. If you are drinking a lot of alcohol, you will want to drink even more water, as alcohol will dehydrate you. If you're not used to drinking this much water, I encourage you start increasing it slowly.

Remember the all-or-nothing attitude? I ask that you don't go from drinking hardly any water, to trying to down eight to twelve cups or more a day, because that is what I've written here. If you're used to drinking only two or three glasses in a day, then bump it up to four or five to start. Do that consistently for a few weeks, and then bump it up again by one or two glasses. Slowly work your way to the eight to twelve average, depending on your body weight, and give your body a chance to adapt. It will be much easier to stick to this habit long-term than if you try to do it all at once. You'll also be running to the washroom so frequently that it may disrupt your daily activities and sleep.

I know that for myself, getting into a steady water drinking routine was one of my biggest challenges. I have some clients who also find it a difficult habit to get into. Here are some water drinking tactics that work for me and could help you too:

- Try to keep a water bottle or large glass handy at your desk, in your car, or anywhere else where you'll be spending a lot of your time over the course of the day. Make sure you keep it within view and reach as a visual reminder. If for example, you know you will be in meetings all day, and all they typically serve is coffee and soft drinks, be sure that you have access to your water bottle and that you fill it up prior to going into your meetings. At break time, be sure to fill it up again, so it is there when you want it.

• If you don't like the taste of plain water, you can always make it more palatable with a twist of lemon or lime. You could also mix it with a bit of 100% fruit juice to give it some flavour.

• Another way to get your water intake is to eat foods with high water content such as juicy fruits and vegetables. Apples, oranges, peaches, watermelon, and grapes are good choices. Lettuce, cucumber, celery, and tomatoes are all great options too.

• Decaffeinated coffee and tea can also be considered part of your water intake. So if you drink three cups of herbal tea a day and one decaffeinated coffee, you'll want to add four to eight cups or more of water to that, depending on your weight and suggested daily requirement.

• Fruit juices are a good choice too, but they are very concentrated sources of calories and natural sugar. A good idea is to dilute them to half juice and half water. This way, you get the taste but only half the sugar and calories per serving.

About Alcohol

If you're used to having a few drinks now and again, take note that alcohol can have an impact on your healthy eating, weight control and positive living results in more ways than one. Alcohol is not only high in calories, it also lowers your resistance to cravings and impulse food choices. You may have a good time in the moment, but remember how your health, weight and lifestyle results will be compromised in the long-run. Alcohol will only help keep the weight on. This is especially true as you age. The harsh truth is that as you get older, your body becomes more sensitive to the effects of alcohol. This even includes red wine, which you may be told is good for you. I ask that for the sake of your health, weight and lifestyle results, you think twice before indulging in your usual amount of alcohol.

Here are some tips on how to start cutting back slowly:

1) Add ice to your glass if you're having white wine.

2) Sip your wine slowly.

3) Or, better yet, have something non-alcoholic instead.

4) If you like beer, then opt for the non-alcoholic option.

If you're used to having two or three glasses of wine in one sitting, then cut it back to one or two, and work your way to only one or two glasses per week at most.

Remember, this isn't just about your weight, it's about your health too. Experts now say that drinking too much alcohol in a woman's menopausal years increases the risk of breast cancer. Is it really worth it?

Gradual Change for Long-Term Results

My clients are always telling me that as they slowly cut back on their less healthy choices, and replace them with higher fibre, lower fat, reduced-sodium, reduced-sugar and reduced-calorie foods, they are amazed that they start to resist the less healthy choices with greater ease, without feeling hungry or deprived. They actually find themselves enjoying their new way of eating. For example, I had one client who loved pizza and made a simple small change from thick crust to thin crust to cut back on the quantity of insulin-boosting white starches. She and her whole family enjoyed it much more. They found they could taste a lot more of the toppings without so much dough. She also noticed that she didn't feel as bloated afterward. She saved herself a number of calories too.

I can remember a time when my automatic coffee drinking habit was with three sugars and three creams. When I decided to take control of my health and weight, I chose to gradually cut back by consciously starting with taking only two sugars and two creams in my coffee. Of course, at first, it didn't taste quite sweet enough or rich enough compared to my usual habit, but it wasn't a huge change. After a short while, I got used to it and my new automatic coffee drinking habit was with two sugars and two creams. Once that became very comfortable for me, and I was no longer missing the extra cream and sugar, I decided to repeat the process. I cut back again, and tried my coffee with only one sugar and one cream. Again, it tasted a bit different from what I was used to, but I persisted and eventually I got to like my coffee with one sugar and one cream. I did it one more time and dropped the one sugar.

So now I take my coffee with only one cream and no sugar. Actually, I only use cream in restaurants. At home I use evaporated milk instead, as it is lower in fat and calories, and still gives it that rich creamy texture. The funny thing is my husband drinks his coffee with three sugars and evaporated milk. One day I took a sip of his coffee and couldn't believe how sweet it was. It tasted awful to me. I couldn't believe that I used to drink my coffee that sweet. It just helped to reconfirm for me that no matter how bad life gets, or what kind of day I had, I will never go back to drinking my coffee that sweet again.

I include this to show you how by consciously changing your habits GRADUALLY, you can actually change your taste for certain less healthy foods. Another personal example of sugar habits, is when I used to drink more alcohol. I used to love having wine coolers, especially during the summer. After starting to cut back more and more on sugar, one day I went to have a cooler after not having had one for some time, and all I could taste was the sugar. It didn't even taste good to me, so I didn't bother finishing it. As I slowly cut back on alcohol and sugar, my desire for them lessened. The conclusion I came to, was that the more you eat or drink something, the more you will crave it. As I started eating more foods from the healthy list, I actually found myself craving those foods increasingly, and the less healthy ones decreasingly. It's been a truly magical transformation, one that I would never have dreamed possible, which is what many of you may be thinking right now. However, myself and my clients can't all be crazy. I'm telling you it works. You just have to keep on trying.

What are your three creams and three sugars? That is, what is it that you eat or drink in excess that is high in fat, sugar, salt and calories that you want to GRADUALLY change for better health and weight control?

_____

_____

_____

_____

_____

_____

Starting this moment, what small change can you make to slowly cut back on the quantities and frequencies with which you consume these items?

_____

_____

_____

_____

_____

_____

_____

Does it take more time, effort and commitment to make more frequent choices from the healthy list than the less healthy list? Perhaps, but mostly it simply takes a little bit more thinking. It means remembering your key health, weight and lifestyle motivators from the beginning of this book. You always have to keep at the back of your mind the WHY of why you want to adopt and maintain healthy eating, weight control and positive living habits to begin with. By remembering your big picture goals, you will have better incentives to resist the less healthy choices, and replace them with healthier ones instead. You'll remember that the more calories you eat and the less you burn through physical activity, the more weight you will gain. Therefore, to slowly cut back on high-calorie foods, you must be conscious of WHY you eat less healthy choices, identify trouble food situations, learn to anticipate them ahead of time, and devise strategies to manage them as best possible. This is a habit you need to get into that I will teach you how to do. It means recognizing the automatic habits that get you into these problem situations to begin with.

The Problem

The problem is that most people who struggle with their weight think of the items on the less healthy list as tasty, feels good, easy, fast, convenient and perhaps even *"forbidden"*, especially when dieting the traditional way. In today's fast-paced society where we are often overwhelmed by our To-Do lists, restaurants, fast foods and pre-packaged foods are a welcome relief from having to plan meals ahead of time and make the effort to prepare them. It's true that planning and preparing healthy meals takes a bit more time and energy, and most of us are simply too tired at the end of a stressful day to give it the proper level of thought and effort it requires.

The question then becomes one of what changes you need to make in your daily routine, so that you will have more time and energy to look after yourself properly. At this point, I'd like to introduce some suggestions that I believe we all need to practice to keep our lives balanced. As you get better at managing your time and energy, you yourself will become less stressed, more balanced and happier. I'd like to talk to you now about the effects of stress, the importance of proper sleep, relaxation, fun and passion.

Get Proper Sleep and Relaxation

When people talk about health and weight control, they always talk about healthy eating and getting plenty of exercise. I would like to add the ingredients of proper sleep and relaxation to that mix. I separate the two because proper relaxation and sleep are not necessarily the same. Sleep is when you go to bed at night, turn off the lights, close your eyes and enter a state of unconsciousness. Your body needs a certain amount and quality of sleep to function properly. You don't need me to tell you that, I'm sure.

How do you feel when you first wake up in the morning?

1) Refreshed and keen to start your day

2) Tired, unrefreshed and wishing you could stay in bed just a little bit longer

If you answered "*1*", then my guess is you got sufficient, good quality sleep the night before. If you answered "*2*", then I suspect that you did not get sufficient, good quality sleep the night before. You may have had enough hours of sleep, but what happens inside your brain and body during those hours may not be as productive and healthful as the person who woke up fully energized. It may also mean that you simply didn't get to sleep long enough.

Good sleep habits are critical to your health and sense of well-being, as the ripple effect from a poor night's sleep can have serious implications. For example, when you don't sleep well, you may drink more coffee than usual to stay awake. Too much caffeine isn't healthy and could cause upset stomach, so what do you do? You reach for the antacids to settle your stomach. You may develop headaches for which you take medications to relieve the pain, which may make you drowsier. You may have trouble concentrating and getting things accomplished. You may become less patient and tolerant of others, and less able to solve problems and manage difficult situations effectively. This could have a ripple effect in your personal and workplace relationships, as your behaviour may not be understood or appreciated by others. This creates additional problems, which creates added stress. When you have more stress, it may be more difficult to sleep well, which feeds right into the continuation of this perpetual cycle. When you're overtired, your body may crave sugar and carbohydrates, sending you straight to the insulin-boosting foods on the less healthy food listing. You want these foods for energy, but because of the effect these foods have on your brain, you'll actually want to eat more of them. Also, because you're so tired, your judgment is impaired and your resistance is weakened. You simply do not have the energy to resist temptation and make good choices. These are just some of the implications of improper sleep. When this is a regular occurrence, it can have a serious impact on your overall quality of life. So if you're having serious sleep problems, you may want to bring them up with a medical professional.

When I talk about proper relaxation, I'm referring to your *"down"* time. With all the thinking you have to do all day in getting your work and chores done and solving problems as they arise, your mental health may need you to take some time out to not think and just *"be"*. It is important to have some mindless time to just *"be yourself by yourself"*. Your down time should be your opportunity to do whatever it is that brings you a sense of peace. This is different for everyone. Here are some ideas of what you might do to come to a sense of calm after a hectic day, without turning to food. Check off the ones that appeal to you.

- ❑ Take a nice hot bubble bath.
- ❑ Take a bath with Epsom salts for added health benefits.
- ❑ Quiet your mind listening to peaceful music.
- ❑ Read a light fiction novel as you don't want to read anything too heavy or upsetting, especially right before bed.
- ❑ Write your thoughts in a personal journal.
- ❑ Put on some music and just dance, moving any which way your body takes you, not caring what you might look like.

- ❑ Go for a walk.
- ❑ Close your eyes, sit or lie down quietly and slow down your breathing.
- ❑ Do something creative that you can lose yourself in completely such as drawing, painting, sculpture, playing a musical instrument or some form of arts and crafts.
- ❑ Do something manual that involves building or repairing something such as building or refinishing a piece of furniture or home improvement.

These are just some suggestions. *What else can you add to this list that you can see yourself realistically doing to slow down, catch your breath and quiet your mind to regain your balance after the activities of the day?*

_____

_____

_____

_____

_____

_____

_____

Incorporate More Fun and Laughter into Your Daily Life

Laughter is a great stress reliever. I truly believe that one of the greatest feelings in the world is to experience fun and laughter, especially the kind of laughter that makes your stomach hurt and brings tears to your eyes. Being able to see the lighter side of life through moments that may otherwise seem very dark, is a gift. Humour is a powerful tool to ease pain. Laughter is what I call a positive high. It is energizing. When you are on a positive high and feeling energized, you are better able to deal with life's daily challenges and the physical effects of stress. When it comes to food choices, the more positive mindset you have, the easier it is to make conscious healthy choices, so keep smiling. Laughter can be contagious. Therefore, I encourage you to surround yourself with people who like to laugh, who make you happy, and who are fun and lively, without the need for copious amounts of alcohol and unhealthy foods.

Avoid Boredom By Finding Your Passion

Passion is a driving life force. When you have interests and activities outside of your work life that you feel passionate about, you are less likely to face boredom. People with many interests and passions rarely get bored, as they can always find something they like to do. This is so important in relation to your eating habits, because when you have interests and passions, you then have something to turn to, other than food, through which to gain comfort and cope with stress. For example, one of my passions is reading books on psychology, health and spirituality. Learning gives me great joy. When I get my hands on a new book that gets me thinking in new and exciting ways, I forget about the world around me and lose all track of time.

What are you interested in or feel passionate about? It could be anything.

_____

_____

_____

_____

_____

_____

_____

How do you think you can use this interest or passion in dealing with challenging food situations?

_____

_____

_____

_____

_____

_____

_____

What will you do differently next time to deal with a difficult food situation?

_____

_____

_____

_____

_____

_____

_____

Let's Give a Hand to Proper Serving Portions

In our society's mindset, where *"bigger is always better"*, many people have completely lost touch with what a normal portion of food actually looks like on their plate. As a result, it has become entirely normal to eat in quantities far greater than what our bodies actually need. This is especially true today, where we live a much more sedentary lifestyle with many more conveniences than before. For example, in the old days, people actually had to get up out of their chairs to turn channels on the television. Can you imagine getting up every time you wanted to change the channel? Or, to use the telephone, people had to get up and go to the one telephone in the house plugged into the wall, whereas now we have our cordless phones and cell phones tied to our hip. They had to walk to the market and carry their bags back home, whereas now we tend to drive everywhere. With modern day drive-throughs, we don't even have to get out of our cars. In the old days, people had to climb stairs, and now we have escalators and elevators to carry us where we want to go.

These are just a few examples. Now we can sit at our computers for hours on end, barely getting up to have something to eat or go to the washroom. We sit and we sit. The more we sit, the more tired we become. Suddenly, any reason to get up can become draining and viewed as an inconvenience. We sit and we sit. We sit in the office and then we sit in the restaurant, where the portions and plate sizes just keep getting bigger and bigger. Then we go home and we sit in front of the television. It's even worse for today's children, who are being raised with computers and video games. It's no wonder that the rate of child obesity is growing at a frightening rate.

The problem is that too many of us grew up in homes where we were programmed by our parents to ALWAYS eat everything on our plate. That's fine when you have a reasonably sized plate filled with a good balance and variety of healthy foods in proper portions. However, when you compare the foods we eat today with those we grew up with, and the serving size expectations as dictated by most restaurants, eating everything on our plate as we've been programmed to do, is actually counterproductive to good health and effective weight control in today's world. Therefore, it is high time to reprogram this habit by learning proper portion sizes and sticking to them regardless of plate size or how much food is on it, whether we're at home, in a restaurant or a guest in someone's home. Eating in restaurants and at social gatherings is a regular occurrence for some more than others. If you tend to eat out or in the company of others fairly often, then the next time you're dining in these potentially difficult food situations, I ask that you consider the following strategies:

1) Avoid arriving over-hungry. If you anticipate lots of food temptations and less healthy food choices, then have a glass of water and a light healthy snack at least thirty minutes before the event. This will help curb your appetite by partially filling your stomach so that you don't risk being famished upon arrival. When you're over-hungry, it's more difficult to step back and make good choices in proper portion sizes. Instead, you may end up eating anything in sight, and then regretting it later.

2) Share your meal.

3) Take home the leftovers. There is nothing wrong with taking home some leftover entrée that was probably big enough to feed at least two.

4) Start your meal with a bowl of non-creamy soup and/or a tossed salad. This will help to fill you up with minimal calories so you don't overeat on the higher calorie main course. It will make it easier to stick to proper serving sizes.

5) When the main course comes, be sure to start with your vegetables, so you fill up on low-calorie items first. Then eat your proper portion of protein. Then eat your proper portion of starch.

6) If the only choices for starches are white rice, French fries or baked potato, consider replacing these choices with extra steamed vegetables or a garden salad instead. If you really want the starch, then choose your portions wisely based on how many servings of other starches you had throughout the day. That is, if you've already

had a lot of starches in your day and hardly any vegetables, then you will definitely want to skip the starch and catch up on your vegetables with a side salad instead.

7) Unless there's a dessert on the menu that is an absolute must-have, avoid dessert completely as the extra sugar, fat and calories are not worth it. If you can't resist temptation, or consciously give yourself permission to have a special dessert, then consider sharing it, or only eating a few bites and taking the rest home for another day.

8) Avoid the white buns and rolls that come to the table. If brown buns or rolls are served, start with only half. You can also ask the server to either not bring them to the table or take them away so they're not in view to tempt you.

9) As it's easy to get caught up in conversation and not realize how much you're eating, try noticing when you're halfway through your meal and put your cutlery down onto the plate. Consciously stop eating for a few minutes to give the food a chance to go down. It takes your brain a good twenty minutes to register that you're full, so if you stop halfway and wait a while, you may not eat as much when you finally do return to eating. Ask yourself if you're really hungry for more, or already satisfied.

Most importantly, you need to learn to respond to your body's real needs. Give it a chance to tell you if it's still hungry or already full.

Get into the habit of feeling satisfied by choosing bigger portions of low-calorie foods such as vegetables, beans, soups, salads, and low-fat dairy, with much lighter portions of anything from the less healthy food list.

In the next section, I will provide you with a table listing the best choices for food groups with proper single serving size and suggested daily number of servings for balanced eating. Since it is not always practical or manageable to weigh your food according to the measurements provided, I will first give you an easy, practical and manageable way to measure all of your food quantities by visually comparing them to your hand. The reason this system worked so well for me, and could work well for you too, is that you carry your hand with you wherever you go. It is a practical, manageable and flexible means for you to gauge the quantities of food you should be eating, without having to measure or weigh your food.

The idea is to eat a balanced variety of foods in the proper portion sizes from each group. As you use the tables more and more, you will start to remember proper portion sizes automatically. They will become part of you, and eventually you will no longer need to turn to the table for reference. However, until then, I suggest keeping a copy of the tables handy at all times for easy reference.

How to Eat in a Balanced Way:
Best Choices for Food Groups with Proper Single Serving Size and Suggested Daily Number of Servings

See tables on the following pages.

*NOTE: serving sizes will vary according to age, gender and activity level. The more active you are, the more you can eat to replenish your energy, as you need ample calorie consumption for sufficient energy to burn. If you are male, you can generally eat more servings than women, as your required calorie intake is slightly higher than for women.

Hand measurement equivalents:

1 cup	=	1 fist
½ cup	=	½ fist
3 ounces	=	1 palm
1 tsp	=	1 thumb tip
1 tbsp	=	2 thumb tips

BREAD	**(Aim for 3-4 daily)** 1 slice brown bread. Compare product labels and select one with 3 grams of fibre or more 1 brown English muffin 2 slices low-calorie bread ½ whole wheat dinner roll ½ whole wheat hamburger or hot dog bun ½ whole wheat bagel ½ whole wheat pita ½ cup cooked brown rice no salt 1 cup whole wheat pasta no salt ½ cup cooked couscous no salt ½ cup cooked bulgar no salt 2 long or 4 short breadsticks (2 grams or less of fat) 25 pretzel sticks 4 no-fat or three low-fat crackers with 2 grams or less of fat and 2 grams of fibre or more) 3 cups air popped popcorn 1 whole wheat flour tortilla ¾ cup low-fat ready-to-eat cold cereal with 2 grams of fat or less and 4 grams or more of fibre per serving. ½ cup cooked hot cereal with 2 grams of fat or less and 4 grams or more of fibre per serving. 1 waffle 1 pancake
VEGETABLE	**(Aim for 3 or more)** 1 cup raw leafy vegetables ½ cup plain (no butter, margarine, oil or sauce added preferably) fresh, frozen, steamed or microwaved. ½ cup canned vegetables rinsed of salt and added sugar ¾ cup vegetable juice ½ cup cooked white or sweet potato no salt
FRUIT	**(Aim for 2-3 daily)** 1 small apple, pear, orange, or other fresh fruit 1 cup fresh strawberries, grapes, cherries, or other berries 1 cup frozen fruits no added sugar or syrup ½ cup fresh fruit salad no added sugar ½ cup canned fruit rinsed of added sugar and syrup ½ cup fresh fruit juice from concentrate no added sugar ¾ ounces dried fruit 1 cup applesauce

MEAT or SUBSTITUTES	**(Aim for 2-4 daily)** 3 ounces of low-fat fish such as cod, halibut, haddock or flounder 3 ounces of fish high in omega-3 fatty acids such as salmon or mackerel ½ cup shrimp or other shellfish ½ cup canned tuna in water ¼ cup canned salmon 5 sardines 3 ounces herring 3 ounces of chicken or turkey breast ½ cup extra lean ground beef, chicken or turkey 2 egg whites (avoid egg yolks as they are high in cholesterol) ¼ cup fat-free egg substitute ½ cup cooked dried beans such as chickpeas, kidney, romano, black beans and other beans. If you use canned beans be sure to rinse thoroughly 3 ounces lean meat with all visible fat removed including pork tenderloin, steak, lamb, veal and other meats 1 egg (avoid eating too many eggs as they are high in cholesterol) 7 cashews, almonds or walnuts, 20 peanuts 2 tablespoon peanut butter *Peanut butter is high in fat so be advised to eat sparingly as a meat substitute*
DAIRY	**(Aim for 2-3 daily)** 1 cup skim milk ½ cup evaporated skim milk 1 cup fat-free soy milk no sugar added ½ cup no-fat no-sugar added yogurt, cottage cheese or quark cheese 4 tbsp no-fat cream cheese, 2 tbsp light cream cheese or 1 tbsp regular cream cheese ½ cup dairy desserts such as no-fat pudding, frozen yogurt or ice cream 1 tbsp feta cheese 1 ounce low-fat hard cheese *If the no-fat option is not available look for products with 2 grams or less of fat per ½ cup serving*
FATS/OILS	**(Eat sparingly – 2-3 daily)** 1 tsp monounsaturated oils such as olive, canola or peanut oil. ¼ avocado 1 tsp butter, margarine, mayonnaise or salad dressing 7 cashews, almonds or walnuts or 20 peanuts *Avoid products with coconut, palm and other tropical oils as much as possible. Be sure to READ YOUR LABELS*

BEVERAGES	(Aim for 8-12 or more cups daily (depending on weight) Add 1 for every 4 ounces of alcohol
	Plain water (minimum 6) Decaffeinated coffee or tea no sugar (no more than 3 total) Fruit or vegetable juice (no more than 1) Diet soda (no more than 1)

EXAMPLE OF A POSSIBLE DAY INTAKE based on Best Choices Table

FOOD INTAKE	SERVINGS	SUBTOTAL FOR DAY	REMAINING PORTIONS FOR DAY
Breakfast			
1 slice high-fibre bread	1 bread	1 bread	2-3 bread
1 tbsp peanut butter	½ meat	½ meat	1½-3½ meat
½ cup strawberries	½ fruit	½ fruit	1½-2½ fruit
½ cup no-fat yogurt	1 dairy	1 dairy	1-2 dairy
		0 fat	2-3 fat
		0 vegetable	3-5 vegetable
1 cup decaffeinated coffee	1 beverage	1 beverage	7-11 beverage
2 cups of plain water (you can add lemon slices to flavour)	2 beverage	3 beverage	5-9 beverage
Mid-morning Snack			
3 low-fat crackers	1 bread	2 bread	1-2 bread
		½ meat	1½-3½ meat
		½ fruit	1½-2½ fruit
1 ounce low-fat hard cheese	1 dairy	2 dairy	0-1 dairy
		0 fat	2-3 fat
½ cup raw vegetables such as carrots, celery or broccoli. *Note that cheese is also high in protein so may also be considered a small meat serving.	1 vegetable	1 vegetable	2+ vegetable
1 cup of plain water (you can add lemon slices to flavour)	1 beverage	4 beverage	4-8 beverage
Lunch			
½ whole wheat bagel	1 bread	3 bread	0-1 bread
½ cup canned tuna	1 meat	1½ meat	½ -2½ meat
		½ fruit	1½-2½ fruit
1 tbsp light cream cheese	½ dairy	2½ dairy	½-1 dairy
2 tsp oil based salad dressing	2 fat	2 fat	0-1 fat
1 cup lettuce greens, ¼ cup tomato ¼ cup chopped red pepper ⅛ cup cucumber & ⅛ cup celery	2 vegetable	3 vegetable	0+ vegetable
1 cup decaffeinated tea	1 beverage	5 beverage	3-7 beverage

EXAMPLE OF A POSSIBLE DAY INTAKE *(continued)*

FOOD INTAKE	SERVINGS	SUBTOTAL FOR DAY	REMAINING PORTIONS FOR DAY
Mid-Afternoon Snack 1 apple ½ cup no fat yogurt	1 fruit 1 dairy	3 bread 1½ meat 1½ fruit 3½ dairy 2 fat 3 vegetable	0-1 bread ½-2½ meat ½-1½ fruit 0 dairy 0-1 fat 0+ vegetable
2 cups of plain water (you can add lemon slices to flavour)	2 beverage	7 beverage	1-5 beverage
Dinner ½ cup cooked brown rice seasoned 6 oz grilled salmon steak ½ cup frozen berries with ¼ cup yogurt	1 bread 2 meat ½ fruit ½ dairy	4 bread 3½ meat 2 fruit 4 dairy 2 fat	0 bread 0-½ meat 0-1 fruit 0 dairy 0-1 fat
1 cup cooked broccoli ½ cup cooked green beans ¼ cup cooked vegetables to mix with rice	3 vegetable	6 vegetable	0+ vegetable
1 cup of plain water (you can add lemon slices to flavour)	1 beverage	8 beverage	0-4 beverage
Evening Snack ½ cup strawberries	½ fruit	4 bread 3½ meat 2½ fruit 2 fat 4 dairy 6 vegetable	0 bread 0-½ meat 0-½ fruit 0-1 fat 0 dairy 0+ vegetable
1 decaffinated tea	1 beverage	9 beverage	0-3 beverage

Summary for Day

FOOD GROUP	SUGGESTED SERVINGS DAILY	ACTUAL SERVINGS
Bread	3-4	4
Vegetables	3 or more	6
Fruit	2-3	2½
Meat	2-4	3½
Dairy	2-3	4
Fats	2-3	2
Beverage	8-12	9

If you look at the example, you'll see that by keeping track of your subtotals as you go along through your day, you'll be better able to make healthy balanced choices at every eating opportunity. By writing it all down, you'll be forced to pay attention to your choices. If for example, by 3:00 p.m. you haven't had any vegetables or dairy, you will want to make sure that your mid-afternoon snack, dinner and evening snacks compensate by including a number of vegetable and dairy servings. If you aim to eat balanced meals and snacks throughout the day, it is easier to get in all your servings. The more you can plan your meals in advance, the better. However, even with the best of intentions, things don't always go smoothly, or you may not have had a chance to plan properly. When this happens, just do the best you can for what's left of the day, making the most balanced choices where possible. Let it go if things get off track and pay attention to the WHY things went awry. Focus on fixing the reasons for WHY things went off track, and decide what you'll do differently next time to avoid similar circumstances.

If you look at the summary table, you can see that this is an example of a good day, as you stayed within the suggested serving guidelines. If you normally eat significantly more than the suggested servings for any particular food group, you'll want to gradually cut back by 1-2 servings for every food group that is above the suggested servings. For example, if you regularly eat the equivalent of 7 or 8 bread servings in a day, then you'll want to start by cutting back to 5 or 6 servings. Stay with that for 2-3 weeks, then cut it back again to 4-5 servings and stick with that for 2-3 weeks, and then cut it back to 3-4 servings daily.

This is a more gradual change that is easier on your body and will make the transition easier for you. It gives you a chance to get used to the new amount. If there are food groups that you are not eating enough of, then you need to gradually increase the number of servings. For example, if you're only eating 1-2 serving of vegetables in a typical day, then increase it to 2-3 servings, stick with that for 2-3 weeks, and then increase it again to 3 or more servings.

Using these examples, you can create your own menu plans for the day, plan your meals ahead of time, or simply keep track on a meal to meal basis. Be sure to do a summary and see how you did. This will help you determine which food groups you need to bump up or down. See the next page for blank sample forms that you can use to keep track.

FOOD INTAKE	SERVINGS	SUBTOTAL	REMAINING
Breakfast			
Beverage			
Mid-morning snack			
Beverage			
Lunch			
Beverage			
Mid-afternoon snack			
Beverage			
Dinner			
Beverage			
Evening snack			
Beverage			

Summary for Day

FOOD GROUP	SUGGESTED SERVINGS DAILY	ACTUAL SERVINGS
Bread	3-4	
Vegetables	3 or more	
Fruit	2-3	
Meat	2-4	
Dairy	2-3	
Fats	2-3	
Beverage	8-12	

The Power of Choice: Moving from Mindlessness to Mindfulness

"By becoming a conscious choice-maker, you begin to generate actions that are evolutionary for you."

- Deepak Chopra

Now that you know how to recognize healthy versus less healthy choices, decide on proper portion sizes, and balance your servings of various food groups for proper nutrition, you now have an incredible power within you – the power of choice. The critical factor, is that from this moment forward, you need to make as many conscious choices, instead of automatic ones, as often as possible. This is something you'll have to do for the rest of your life, in order to maintain the positive changes in habit you develop. After all, it is your automatic choices that got you into trouble in the first place. By learning to awaken to your choices in the moment they present themselves, you have the power to now be *in control of* your eating rather than be *controlled by* your eating.

Here's another way to think of it. Imagine that you've always driven cars with automatic transmissions. The car automatically shifts gears for you, so you don't even have to think about it. All you do is put your foot on the gas and go. This is the only *"automatic"* driving habit you've ever known. Now imagine that you're given a brand new sports car, the car of your dreams, but it has a manual transmission instead of automatic. Suddenly, you can't just push on the gas and go. You now have to learn a whole new way to drive. You need to pay attention to the sounds of the engine as the RPM increases, and know when to shift gears up and down. It may be awkward at first. You may have trouble shifting smoothly from one gear to the next. However, with practice it will get easier and easier to the point where shifting becomes second nature.

Now think of this car as your body. You're used to feeding it mindlessly. I am now asking you to take your foot off the gas pedal and get out of automatic mode. You need to start listening to the sound of your own engine and know when and how to smoothly shift gears. This means noticing what you're doing, as in knowing when to give gas and when to let go, so to speak. At first it may seem awkward and you'll have to concentrate hard to make the right decisions. Over time and with practice, it will become easier and easier.

Even now, after reaching and maintaining my healthy weight, I still must consciously choose my foods and portion sizes, and do a constant mental check throughout the day to make sure I'm eating as balanced as possible. I still have to listen to my body, know when to switch gears, and give it just the right amount of fuel it requires.

What really worked for me, was to constantly remind myself of the following wisdom. I ask that you adopt this same wisdom and allow it to work for you too.

With every choice I make, in any given moment, comes a personal sacrifice and a personal gain. I know this to be true not only for my food choices, but for every decision I will ever make in life.

These words apply to both your healthy and less healthy food choices. For example, if you make a healthy choice, such as an apple over your favourite, less healthy one, such as chocolate cake or a bag of potato chips, then the personal sacrifice is the instant taste-satisfaction, reward and comfort that your favourite, more automatic choice would have given you. The personal gain derived by eating the apple instead, is better weight management, minimized health risks, greater self-esteem and happiness. Wouldn't you agree that the personal gain far outweighs the sacrifice in the long-run? The problem is that we don't tend to think about what's best for us in the long-run, when faced with that rich chocolate cake or salty bag of chips. All we typically think about is the here and now, forgetting the emotional pain that these instant gratification choices will cause us soon after.

On the flip side, if you choose to eat the chocolate cake or bag of chips instead of the apple, then the personal sacrifice is increased risk of weight gain, associated health risks, lowered self-esteem and happiness. The only personal gain is the instant gratification and comfort that lasts only moments. Here the gain DOES NOT outweigh the sacrifice, so you're much better off to stick to healthier choices and proper portion sizes for every aspect of your health – physical, mental, emotional and spiritual. Remember, it is all about choices. You have the power of choice, so use that power wisely. The challenge in these instances is to decide whether the temporary pleasure of taste and comfort is worth the long-term pain of your diminished health and self-esteem.

The same goes for exercise. If you choose to incorporate more physical activity into your daily routine, then the personal sacrifice is NOT doing what you may rather be doing instead, or that you may deem more important. The personal gain is healthy weight control, a higher fitness level, more muscle tone, more energy, a stronger and leaner body, healthier cardiovascular system, increased self-esteem and more positive body-image. Let me ask you, does the personal gain of doing the exercise not far outweigh the personal sacrifice? If you choose NOT to exercise, then your personal sacrifice includes continued weight problems, lowered fitness level, less muscle tone accompanied by more body fat, less energy, a less healthy cardiovascular system, lowered self-esteem, negative body-image and greater weight-related health risks. Again, the personal gain of exercise far outweighs the personal sacrifice. The choice is YOURS alone to make. It is all about remembering and reconnecting to what is truly most important to you in the grand scheme of things.

Playing the FREEZE Game

Now that you understand the theory of personal gain vs. personal sacrifice, and short-term pleasure vs. long-term pain, I want to present you with some questions to help you challenge and conquer your automatic self-sabotaging self-talk. The key is not only to memorize these questions, but to also remember to use them as consistently as possible.

First, here is a tip for you. Remember when you were a kid and you played a game called *"FREEZE"*? Perhaps you had a few friends over, sitting around the kitchen table having a snack, and someone suddenly yelled out the word *"FREEZE"*. The idea of the game was to freeze your body no matter what position you were in and not move again for as long as you can. The first person to move was the loser. When you are in a difficult food situation, and about to eat a questionable choice or portion size, I ask that you pretend you're playing the *"FREEZE"* game. Before you sink your teeth into it mindlessly out of automatic habit, pretend that someone yelled out *"FREEZE"*. Then, in your mind's eye, step outside of yourself and look at what you're about to eat.

This is your moment of choice. This is when you need to remember WHY you want to shed your unwanted pounds so badly. This is the moment you need to remember how you felt about yourself when you last looked in the mirror, or saw yourself in a photograph. Remember how you felt when you last went shopping for clothes and couldn't find anything that fit properly. Remind yourself of how you feel when you have no energy throughout your day. This is the moment to remember the weight-related health problems you're either fighting or trying to avoid. This is the moment to ask yourself the following questions. Memorize these questions. Keep a copy of these questions handy for easy reference. Post a copy on the fridge or keep it in a kitchen drawer, another copy in your place of work and in your car, or in your purse or wallet, as friendly reminders. One of the first habits you need to develop is to *"FREEZE"* and ask yourself the following questions. By simply asking the very first of the questions, you will immediately be taken out of your automatic mode and into self-awareness. It is only by waking up and taking notice that you can exercise your true power of choice.

Questions to WAKE UP and TAKE NOTICE:

1) *What is it that I'm about to eat?*
2) *Is this a healthy or less healthy choice?*
   - For example, think about the sugar, fat, salt, fibre and calorie content.

If it is a healthy choice, then ask yourself the following:

1) *Is it a balanced choice?*
2) *What is a proper portion size?*
3) *How much of it will I choose to eat?*

If it is a less healthy choice, then ask yourself the following:

1) *"Why am I choosing to consume this when I know it is not a best choice?"*

Here are some possible answers with insights to help you question your decision and start making smarter choices.

I am choosing to consume this because:

"I'm hungry."

My rationale is that if you're genuinely hungry, in that your body needs fuel to support itself, then by all means eat something. However, you still have the power of choice. Be sure to reach for something healthy that will satisfy you. Avoid letting yourself go without food for too long where you end up feeling ravenous and desperate to eat. This will put you at greater risk of making poor food choices and wanting to eat anything and everything in sight.

"It tastes good."

This is what I've concluded to be the number one reason why it's so hard to lose weight and keep it off. The problem is that food DOES taste good, and that's not going to change. The only other thing in the equation is YOU. Therefore, YOU are the one who must change.

"It's in front of me."

If you tend to grab food automatically because it's *"there"*, either put the food out of sight, or move yourself away from it so you don't see it. If you and your family are in the habit of leaving less healthy food choices around on the counters or coffee table in your home, then get everyone to agree to keep these out of sight. Put them away as soon as you use them. Typical foods that people have lying around in plain view are chips, nuts, cookies and other snack foods. If you don't see them, you may not think about them.

"It's a habit."

Just because it's a habit now, doesn't mean you have to give in to it. Remember, you are trying to break unhealthy habits. Now is the time to start. Remember to think about WHY you want to break these habits to begin with. Think about what you can do differently that you would be more proud of.

"It's fast, easy or convenient."

Fast, easy and convenient doesn't mean you have to make poor choices. If fast, easy and convenient is important to you, then learn how to make *"healthy"* foods fit the bill. For example, you're at work and craving sweets. You head for the vending machine to buy your favourite chocolate bar. Now you're not only wasting calories, but money too. Save calories and money by bringing healthy snacks from home to keep in your desk drawer. You're much better off to have a fruit or small quantity of dried fruit instead. Or if you really want that chocolaty taste, have a few spoonfuls of a low-fat chocolate pudding.

"I'm too tired or lazy to prepare something healthy."

Perhaps you had a hard day or didn't sleep well the night before. Your energy is low. It's dinner time and you want to order your family's favourite high-calorie, high-salt, high-fat pizza. Instead of giving in to this temptation every time, you could cook food in larger batches and freeze leftovers in serving size containers. This way, when you're too tired or lazy to cook something healthy, all you have to do is defrost it and presto, you have an instant meal. The work has already been done when you did manage to cook something.

"It's what is expected of me (i.e. in social situations)."

A perfect example is at birthdays and holidays. At birthdays you're always expected to have birthday cake and ice cream. How many times do you eat it just out of obligation, because it's what is expected of you? You are more than likely already full and satisfied from a wonderful birthday meal, but when that magical birthday cake comes out, you wouldn't even dream of not having any. Christmas is another dangerous time when you might eat choices and portion sizes because it is *"tradition"*, and what's expected of you. You'll have to learn to assert yourself and do things differently in these situations. I had one client who was thrilled after gaining 3 lbs over Christmas. I asked her why she was so happy. She said it was because the previous year she had put on 12 lbs over Christmas. She only gained 3 lbs because she made smarter choices that were right for her.

"I can't say no."

Really? You really can't say no? Who said so? Remember you CAN say no. It's your choice. If you continue to say to yourself *"I can't say no"*, then you'll keep on doing whatever necessary to prove yourself right. I am asking you to challenge yourself, and do what's needed to prove to yourself that *"I CAN say no"* instead.

"It's my reward after a particularly stressful or good experience."

Listen to yourself when you say this, and hear how illogical it really is. Rewarding yourself with less healthy food choices that will give you that instant sense of comfort, relief and satisfaction will only cause you greater emotional pain next time you face yourself in the mirror, get on the scale, or visit your doctor only to find out you have developed a weight-related health problem such as diabetes or heart disease. It doesn't make good sense. Be smarter about your choices and find other ways to reward yourself that don't involve food.

"I don't care. I just want it. I'll make up for it tomorrow."

When you hear this type of counterproductive self-talk setting in, challenge it and conquer it. Don't allow it to take control of you. Yes, of course you want it, but is it really true that you don't care? My guess is you really do care. This type of attitude can throw you off track and it may be harder to make healthier choices the next day. If you absolutely must have it, then at least choose your portion size wisely and balance it with smarter picks the rest of your day and week.

"I already had something bad today so my day is already shot. May as well have it and worry about the consequences later."

This is the *"all-or-nothing"* attitude we discussed earlier. Be very careful of this type of thinking. Just because you may have made a mindless choice in the morning that you aren't particularly proud of, does not mean that your whole day is shot. Recognize that you did it, let it go, and plan on what you'll do differently the next time you're faced with a similar food trigger or situation. I ask that you let go of what you did earlier in the day, and focus on getting back on track at the very next meal or snack.

"I'm feeling angry, sad, lonely, anxious or bored and I know that eating this choice is the only thing that will make me feel better."

Is eating REALLY the only thing that can possibly make you feel better? Perhaps that is what your habit is and what you believe to be true, but I ask that you start challenging this belief. Next time you feel this way, try to change your behaviour instead. Do something else, other than eat, to distract you and take your mind off of your problems and your food.

What other reasons can you think of why you may want to eat or drink something that you know is not a best choice?

_____

_____

_____

_____

_____

_____

_____

2) **"Is the short-term pleasure worth the long-term pain? Is it worth it?"**

The underlying question here is *"Are the few moments of TASTE, COMFORT and SATISFACTION really worth the self-sabotage of my LONG-TERM proper eating, healthy weight control and positive living goals?"*

Again, this is the crucial moment where you need to take that step back and remind yourself WHY you want to take control of your eating, weight and lifestyle to begin with. Think about what being healthy and fit will mean for you in the bigger picture. For example, if you want to eat healthy and manage your weight to feel better, look better, have more energy, more confidence or an easier time shopping for clothes, then the next time you're faced with one of your favourite sweets, snacks or other comfort food, ask yourself what is most important to you? Is the immediate in-the-moment gratification of eating this choice worth the setback it presents to achieving your long-term healthy weight and lifestyle goals?

Think about how important it is to you to feel better, have more energy, or feel better about your health and self-image. Think about how feeling better and having more energy will change your life. Think about the pain you feel when you look in the mirror, see yourself in photographs or have trouble doing simple movements that would be so much easier if you were lighter.

You need to bring that emotional pain and your desire to be rid of it into the present moment, for when you forget about that pain, it is too easy to give in to temptation. If you take a step back from the present moment, think about your desired future, and still CHOOSE to eat the whole bag of chips, then remember that it was YOUR choice. You had the option of foregoing immediate gratification but CHOSE not to in that instant. I ask that you do not expect yourself to be perfect ALL the time. Even if you ate the whole bag of chips fully aware that it is completely counterproductive to your long-term health and weight control goals, this does not mean that you are a failure. Changing your habits is NOT easy and it takes practice like anything else.

Maybe next time you will be stronger and choose differently by either eating only half the bag, a handful or, better yet, none at all, and eat something healthy instead. Remember, this is NOT a diet. It is not as if this is the last time you'll ever eat your favourite comfort food. You can have it again. With regular dieting, you may want to eat your favourite treat in big quantities because you don't know when the next time will be that you eat it. I'm suggesting that you forget this way of thinking. Look at where it's gotten you. When you really crave something, give yourself permission to have it on occasion in a limited quantity, enjoy it, and move on. This is much more realistic for long-term success. I ask that you please be patient and forgiving with yourself. Don't give up. Playing the *"FREEZE"* Game and asking the WAKE UP and TAKE NOTICE questions will give you the power of choice. When you start to have small successes, you will slowly build your confidence and it will get easier and easier to assess the situation and make a healthier choice.

If you decided that the short-term pleasure is not worth the long-term pain, then you have a new decision to make. The next question to ask yourself will determine what action you will take, based on your answers to the first two questions. It is as follows:

3) *"What can I do differently than I would normally? What would constitute a success, no matter how small, that I can feel proud of at the end of the day?"*

The reason I ask you to think of what small change you can make that you can feel proud of, is because too often we tend to over-focus on the negative and not appreciate the positive things we do. Every small success can be a motivator towards bigger successes, so start making small changes and notice the positives.

Here are some possible answers:

"I could have the less healthy choice that I truly want, but only eat or drink a fraction of what I would normally eat or drink, and then fill up any remaining hunger with healthy choices."

For example, if you really want potato chips and your usual habit is to eat a large bag, a first small success would be to leave some chips in the bag. If you're still not satisfied, you could think of healthy substitutes that will fill the gap. Many of my clients use plain popcorn as a healthier substitute. If you're used to eating a whole bag, then even leaving the smallest quantity behind is a first success and one to be very proud of. Over time, you could challenge yourself to start leaving more and more in the bag, and having more and more popcorn to compensate. Popcorn is a great substitute for potato chips because it is still crunchy, but much healthier with less fat, less salt, fewer calories and more fibre, assuming you don't add any butter or salt. Eventually, you may find that you want the chips less and less and actually crave the healthier popcorn choice instead. Remember my coffee drinking example? This same strategy of slowly cutting back applies.

"I could avoid the less healthy choices completely by walking away and doing something else other than eat."

Think about your interests and passions, or do something around the house that you've been putting off. This way you'll not only save calories, you'll also feel good about getting something finished you may not have done otherwise. Do something physical and you can even burn some extra calories.

"I could make only healthy choices instead and enjoy the sense of accomplishment for having taken the harder road."

When you start having small successes, your resolve will become stronger and it will become easier to make healthy choices on a more consistent basis. When you crave potato chips and decide to have a bowl of popcorn instead without feeling deprived, this will give you a great sense of accomplishment that will not only yield greater results, but keep you motivated to keep making these positive choices.

The secret to proper eating, healthy weight management and positive living is to consistently do a mindful check and balance between your healthy and less healthy choices. This means being aware of what you're eating and in what portion sizes ALL the time. This is a big commitment. It takes discipline and energy. One method that helps most people is to keep a daily diary of everything you eat and drink and at what times. It is also important to recognize your various food habits and emotional triggers when something sends you reaching for less healthy choices, especially when you lose control of the quantities that you're eating. What are those triggers and what can you do differently to cope in other ways than with food? Or at least, if you are going to reach for food as a coping mechanism, how can you make healthier conscious choices versus less healthy unconscious choices, and not allow yourself to fall completely off track?

Keeping a Food Diary

See the following sample Daily Food Diary (pages 131, 132). Notice that it doesn't only ask for what you ate and drank. You need to also write down your successes, challenges, exercise, beverage intake, sleep quality and overall feeling for the day. Take notice of the patterns that emerge over the next few weeks. See where your biggest challenges are and work on them. Notice your biggest successes and aim to have more and more of those.

Take note of when you ate, where you are when you're eating, who you're with, what else you're doing at the same time, and why you're eating. You may notice that you tend to have the same kinds of cravings at the same times of day. You may find yourself in challenging food situations with some people more than others. You may see that you are often not eating out of hunger, but for a variety of emotional reasons. Perhaps you're overeating at night time because you didn't eat enough during the day. Or maybe you're not drinking enough water. Perhaps you notice that you run into most of your challenges eating while watching television. I ask that you complete this diary daily for a minimum of six consecutive weeks. I know it's just one more thing to add to your To-Do list, but remember the personal gain vs. personal sacrifice theory? Yes, you may have other things that you either need to get done or would rather be doing than filling out this form, but remind yourself constantly why you want to shed your unwanted pounds and keep them off. Remember the image you have of how much better your life will be, and how great you will feel two years from now, once you've shed your unwanted weight and are keeping it off. Keep your diary. Notice the patterns. Recognize where you need to make changes and start making them TODAY.

TODAY'S DATE: _____

	BREAKFAST	SNACK	LUNCH	SNACK	DINNER	SNACK
What did I eat & drink?						
What time?						
Where was I?						
Who was I with?						
What else was I doing? (i.e. watching television, reading, talking, etc.)						
Why did I eat or drink? (i.e. hungry, bored, habit, stressed, lonely, comfort, reward, social, etc.)						

Total portions of Bread _____ Meat _____ Dairy _____ Fruits _____ Vegetables _____ Fats _____

Total water consumed _____ Coffee _____ Tea _____ Alcohol _____ Soft Drinks _____ Other _____

Exercise for today:

Describe my night's sleep:

Describe my overall feeling for the day:

(Chart continued on next page)

(Chart continued from previous page)

	BREAKFAST	SNACK	LUNCH	SNACK	DINNER	SNACK
Successes: What did I do differently that I am proud of?						
Challenges: What will I do differently next time?						

Here is a wonderful poem about habit. Unfortunately, I have yet to find the name of the author.

Habit

I am your constant companion,
I am your greatest helper or heaviest burden.
I will push you onward or drag you down to failure.
I am completely at your command.
Half the things you do might just as well turn over to me
and I will be able to do them quickly and correctly.

I am easily managed -
you must merely be firm with me.
Show me exactly how you want something done
and after a few lessons, I will do it automatically.
I am the servant of all great people;
and alas, of all failures as well.
Those who are great,
I have made great.
Those who are failures,
I have made failures.

I am not a machine,
though I work with all the precision of a machine
plus the intelligence of a human.
You may run me for a profit or run me for ruin -
it makes no difference to me.

Take me,
train me,
be firm with me,
And I will place the world at your feet.
Be easy with me,
and I will destroy you.

WHO AM I?

I AM HABIT.

- Author unknown

"A" Principle #5:
Activity

This section is about the importance of activity in controlling your weight and improving your quality of life. Of course, when we talk about healthy weight management and positive lifestyle, everyone automatically thinks of activity in terms of physical activity. And yes, I too, address the importance of physical activity. However, some of the major food triggers are boredom, anger, loneliness, stress, frustration, celebration and reward. Physical activity is one way to cope with the emotions that cause these food triggers. That is, when you exercise regularly, you release endorphins that help to alleviate pain, control appetite, provide energy and lift your mood, all helping to manage daily challenges more effectively and minimize the physical effects of stress. Increased endorphin levels have also been said to help women decrease the incidences and severity of hot flashes due to menopause. This will help keep women in a more positive state of mind, allowing for better life management. However, physical activity is not the only activity that can be helpful. Positive mental activity and emotional activity are also key to alleviating the negative feelings that can make you want to turn to food for comfort and solace. In this section, we will look at the importance of each of these types of activity, and how you can incorporate them into your daily life for greater overall health, well-being and happiness.

Physical Activity

I ask that you read this chapter, whether exercise is part of your regular routine or not. If it is part of your life, then this will help reassure you that you are doing the right thing, and may encourage you to rethink your exercise routine. If it is NOT part of your routine, you will want to pay close attention to this section to understand why it is such an important aspect of your new approach to your health, weight and life-style management plan, and how to incorporate it into your daily life.

Why Is Physical Activity So Important?

Physical activity is an important ingredient for permanent healthy weight control and positive living. What many dieters and healthy lifestyle seekers experience when they follow a restrictive food plan without exercise, is a sense of great joy and accomplishment when they see the numbers going down on the scale, and feel their clothes getting looser. Others start to notice their weight change and give them all sorts of compliments. It feels great and encourages them to continue losing weight. The problem in this scenario, is that without regular exercise, while they are shedding excess fat, they are also losing healthy muscle mass. Lean muscle mass increases your metabolism, burns more calories than fat, and helps you move with greater ease and become stronger. Lean muscle also takes up less space than fat, giving you a more toned appearance. There-fore, what you should be aiming for is building and maintaining lean muscle mass while simultaneously changing your eating habits.

If you have lost a lot of weight in the past by drastic dieting with little to no exercise, and then gained it all back and more, you have actually put yourself behind the eight ball in terms of your next attempt at weight reduction. The problem is that when you've lost all that weight, you've not only lost fat, but lean muscle mass too. When you put all the weight back on, it did not come back in the form of lean muscle, but rather as fat, so what you've actually done is slow down your metabolism and increase your fat to muscle ratio. You now have more fat compared to lean muscle than when you started your drastic diet plan. This means that you now have to work even harder to shed the weight than you did previously, because you have even less healthy calorie-burning muscle mass than you did before.

If this sounds discouraging, I ask you to let go of that feeling. Accept it as reality, and simply vow to yourself that you will put a stop to this counterproductive cycle as of TODAY. If you allow it to continue, then you are just hurting yourself in the long-run. If your only motivation for weight reduction is to look better in a pair of jeans, then losing weight by dieting without exercising will help you reach that goal. However, that goal is very superficial and temporary. You will only be able to maintain that weight temporarily if you end up going back to your old eating habits and slowing down your metabolism with the associated loss in muscle. The next thing you know, you will be putting back the weight and having to buy new pairs of jeans in increasingly bigger sizes. Is that really what you want? Is the short-term results of fitting into the smaller size jeans really worth it if you're going to end up back into the larger size jeans or even bigger in no time?

Instead of strictly your appearance, I urge you to make your primary motivators your health, happiness and quality of life. When health is your primary motivator, you will be more likely to make better decisions and maintain positive results. When your looks are motivating you more than your health, then you are at higher risk to shed weight using methods that will only hurt your health in the long-run like dangerous pills, starvation, bulimia or other life-threatening tactics. Again, it will not only hurt you physically, but the mental, emotional, and spiritual discouragement, sense of failure, frustration and distress will become increasingly difficult to overcome with every cycle of weight loss and weight gain that you allow to continue. It is so important that you let go right now of the idea of losing weight by dieting alone. This does not mean that you have to become a muscle bound exercise guru. This does not mean that you have to spend hours at the gym. All it means is that you change your thinking about exercise. It means giving it a fresh new chance and opening yourself up to possibilities. It means trying new things and finding physical activities that you enjoy and feel good about. It means sticking to it long enough to see and feel the results, and not giving up when it just seems too hard.

Getting Into an Exercise Routine

When it comes to doing exercise, most of us understand the value of it in terms of our health and overall sense of well-being. However, we can think of a million excuses NOT to do it. Exercise takes time and energy. It is that one more thing on our To-Do list that we often don't have time or energy for at the end of the day. It never seems to be that high on our priority list, as there are always so many other things we feel we should be doing instead. It is YOU who decides what you could and should be doing and nobody else. It is for this reason that I am here to challenge you. I'm here to make you face those excuses, challenge them and obliterate them from your self-talk.

Let's start off by answering a few questions to help you determine your attitudes toward exercise, and see where your strengths and areas for improvements may lie.

Desired Benefits

All of the following are benefits that can be derived from regular physical activity. Which of the following benefits are most important to you, that you feel can be derived by increasing your level of activity? Put a number beside each one in the order of importance to you, with number 1 being the most important and number 14 being the least important.

_____ Minimize weight-related health risks such as heart disease, diabetes, high cholesterol, high blood pressure and some forms of cancer.

_____ Increase my metabolism.

_____ Firm up and get in shape.

_____ Feel better.

_____ Have more energy.

_____ Increase my muscle strength and flexibility.

_____ Keep my weight under control.

_____ Reduce my symptoms of menopause.

_____ Help me manage stress.

_____ Relieve my anxiety and depression.

_____ Increase my circulation.

_____ Improve my appearance.

_____ Enhance my self-confidence.

_____ Other: _____

Which of the following statements best describes your current regular exercise routine? Check only one.

❏ I exercise a minimum of three times a week aerobically through walking or another form of cardiovascular exercise, and two times minimum a week lifting weights and building muscle strength.

❑ I exercise less than one or two times a week.

❑ I get no exercise at all.

If you answered anything other than *I exercise a minimum of three times a week aerobically through walking or another form of cardiovascular exercise and two times minimum a week lifting weights and building muscle strength,* then you need to look at how to incorporate more physical activity into your routine. When your cardiovascular system, circulatory system and muscles are unchallenged, they become lazy and don't work as efficiently as needed to maintain optimal health and weight. When your body isn't functioning optimally, especially combined with your poor eating habits, you're more likely to: feel tired, have aches and pains in your joints, neck and back; experience more headaches and muscle tension; and as a result, simply not be able to move freely and enjoy life to the fullest. You're limiting your life. The way you feel without exercise becomes your norm. That is, you actually get so used to living with your physical limitations that you can barely imagine what life would be like if you could be free of them.

I'm here to help you see that what is normal for you now may seem easier and more comfortable to live with, but if you could just push yourself beyond your comfort zone long enough to see and feel the benefits, you'll be surprised at how quickly your comfort zone will expand, and your waist shrink. You'll be amazed at how what was normal for you before, will become unacceptable to you, as you become stronger, healthier and more caring and nurturing toward yourself. Your body will look and feel better, you'll be more confident within your appearance and life coping abilities, you'll have a sense of accomplishment that is far greater and more invigorating than the laziness and sense of failure and disappointment that has become your norm. What is normal for you today is not the way it has to be forever. It is simply your starting point or launch pad to a newer you.

One of the challenges to get moving out of your comfort zone is that it takes time and energy. However, most of us feel that when it comes to exercise, we rarely have the time, and when we do have the time, we often are too tired. The irony of it all is that when you increase your exercise, you have more energy, and when you have more energy, you can be more active. The problem is that when you're tired, you don't FEEL like moving or doing exercise. It's much easier to just plop on the couch in front of the television, or go for a power snooze. That is totally understandable. However, there are lots of things in life as an adult that we do regardless of whether we FEEL like doing them or not. You may not FEEL like making your bed in the morning, doing your laundry or even cooking a nutritious meal for yourself and your family, but as a mature adult who looks after yourself and your loved ones, and who wants to be a good role model for your children and others, you will eventually have to do these things whether you FEEL like it or not.

Often times we don't FEEL like doing things simply because we don't have the energy or motivation. We're *"too tired"*, we tell ourselves. In all reality, yes, you may be tired, but if you are honest with yourself, you may also find that you've become lazy. You need to stop permitting yourself to use the *"I'm too tired"* and *"I don't feel like it"* excuses, or any of the other excuses/reasons you use for not exercising. These are the beliefs about yourself which you have programmed in your mind to be true. Well, here again, the only person who makes these beliefs true for you are YOU. You have the power within yourself to change these beliefs. It first starts with acknowledging these excuses and challenging their validity.

If I were to ask WHY you DO NOT exercise a minimum of three times a week aerobically through walking or another form of cardiovascular exercise, and two times minimum a week lifting weights and building muscle strength, which of the following might you answer?

I don't exercise as regularly as I need to for optimal health and weight maintenance because...

    ❑ I don't have time. There's too much else to do.
    ❑ I'm too tired. I have no energy.
    ❑ I'm too lazy.
    ❑ It's so boring.
    ❑ It's too hard.
    ❑ I'm not good at anything physical.
    ❑ I hate sweating.
    ❑ I'm too ashamed of my appearance to work out in public.
    ❑ I'm afraid of injuring myself.
    ❑ I have too many physical restrictions.
    ❑ I can never stick to anything.
    ❑ I have nobody to exercise with.

What other reasons might you have for not exercising regularly?

_____

_____

_____

_____

_____

_____

Each of your excuses comes from what you've come to believe exercise means for you. Your attitude toward physical activity is what's preventing you from embracing it into your life. If you think about the mental attitudes we discussed in Principle #2, you'll see that these same mental attitudes could be preventing you from embracing physical activity into your regular routine. I understand this because I struggled with similar attitudes myself. Perhaps you can relate to my story.

Exercise never came easily to me. All through elementary and high school, gym class was my least favourite. I always felt incompetent, uncoordinated, uncool and out of shape compared with the other kids, especially when it came to anything involving running or team sports. To me, gym class was a waste of time. I found it boring and hard. I also hated to sweat. I would have much rather spent that time drawing and painting, which were activities much more enjoyable to me and within my comfort zone. The only physical activity I truly enjoyed as a child was dancing, but somehow dancing was seldom a big part of gym class.

As I grew up, exercise continued to be something that was of little interest to me, perhaps because I never felt particularly good at it, and it was not a priority in my upbringing. My parents were not involved in any sport or formal exercise routine, and it was simply not emphasized as a priority. Growing up, it was much more important to do well in school, study hard and get good grades than do team sports. I also could never stick to any type of exercise routine long enough to really notice all of its benefits. Regular exercise required a certain level of self-discipline that I always seemed to lack. For people who like routine and have an innate sense of self-discipline, regular exercise may be much easier to manage.

However, if you're like me, who hates routine and lacks self-discipline, then incorporating physical activity into your daily life may be more of a challenge.

What I've learned through personal experience and the experience of my clients, is that sometimes it is imperative to extend ourselves beyond our comfort zones and what comes naturally. In order to do what we know is best for us, we sometimes have to push ourselves beyond our self-imposed beliefs and limitations. This can seem daunting at first, but it does get easier.

When I finally decided to take back control of my health and weight, I forced myself to exercise and had to push myself many times at first when I really didn't FEEL like doing it. I experimented with working out at different times of day with a variety of activities and exercise equipment. Over time, and keeping at it, I learned that for me what works best is to work out first thing in the morning. If I didn't do it first thing in the morning, the likelihood that I would fit it in later in the day grew less and less as the day marched on. Perhaps this is true for you too.

Here's a great analogy that really helped me to put things into proper perspective when it comes to fitting exercise into my day. It has been helpful for many of my clients too, who suffer from the same challenges as me when it comes to the consistent self-discipline and self-motivation required to make exercise a regular part of daily life. I went to a seminar about financial planning. What does financial planning have to do with exercise, you might ask? Well, let me explain. For your financial health and well-being, it is recommended that every time you get money coming in, you immediately take 10% off the top and put it away in a savings or investment account, then, you pay your bills from the money that is left over. Most people will do this the other way around. They will first pay the bills and then, if there is any left over at the end of the day, they will put it into their savings or spend it, yet somehow there is seldom any left over. Funny how that works. So I started to follow this advice and have been putting away 10% of all my income as an investment for my future financial health and security. It made sense to me and I found the self-discipline to make this happen with my finances.

I decided to apply the same approach to my health and exercise. What I used to do is perhaps similar to what many of you are doing now. I used to go about my day doing the things that needed to get done, and if I had time and energy at the end of the day, I would try to squeeze in a few minutes of exercise. And, of course, what usually happened is that by the end of the day, I could find a million excuses NOT to exercise. I didn't have time. I was too tired. I had other commitments, and there you have it, another day would go by with little to no exercise. And once again, I was disappointed in myself, proving myself right that I was just not one of *"those"* people who had the discipline to exercise regularly. This way of thinking clearly was not working for me. I knew I had to amend my attitude, or nothing was going to change, and I would continue to put on weight.

I thought to myself, that if I had the self-discipline and motivation to take 10% off the top from my income to put aside for my future financial wealth, then why could I not apply that same self-discipline and motivation to take 10% off the top of my time and energy each day to put aside for my future physical, mental and emotional health? After all, what would having all this money in the future really mean if I was not healthy or physically fit enough to truly enjoy it? Wasn't the time and effort I was to put into exercise an investment in my future, as well?

With this new perspective, I decided that the only way I could make it happen was to wake up earlier and invest a minimum of 30 minutes of time into exercise. That way it was done, and I had the rest of the day to do all the other things on my To-Do list. I simply chose to make exercise a higher priority on my priority list. Eventually, my 30-minute workout turned into 45 minutes, and now I make it a priority to get a minimum of 60 minutes of exercise into my day, at least four times per week. I started really slowly with cardiovascular activities to get my heart rate up and give my lungs a workout, lifting light weights and doing strengthening exercises on the floor and with an exercise ball. With time, as I could feel my workouts getting easier and easier, I would bump up my level of effort to challenge myself and create different routines to keep it interesting and not get bored, as had typically happened with my earlier fitness attempts.

To this day, I am so proud of myself every single time I complete a workout because I know how hard I had to work to get to this point. I have no intention of becoming muscle bound. I simply want to maintain good health with a healthy heart and lungs, good circulation, flexibility and strong muscle tone. I have no intention of winning competitions. I simply want to feel strong, healthy and confident within my own body. What motivates me to continue with the exercise is that I want to maintain my health, energy, size and healthy weight, and be able to eat my favourite treats now and again guilt-free. All I have to do is look at my *"before"* photo (see page 205), and remind myself that I never want to go back to looking and feeling the way I did when that *"before"* photo was taken.

Exercising makes me feel good about myself, helps me manage stress better, and improves my quality of sleep. With regular exercise, I suffer less headaches, muscle tension and have fewer aches and pains in my neck and back. I also know that when in good shape, your body can heal more quickly from surgeries or injuries. Having survived a car accident at a time when I was not in such great shape, I already know how long it can take to heal injured muscles and ligaments. My husband, who was also in the car accident, was in great physical condition at the time and suffered far less with a much faster rate of healing. You never know what's around the corner, so being in good shape can only help you overcome unforeseen physical problems such as the ones I suffered in my car accident.

So how does all this pertain to you and your attitudes toward exercise? Let me explain. By sharing some insights into my story, I am asking you to reflect on what your story is, as it pertains to your attitudes and challenges in relation to exercise.

Before we go to the next step, I ask that you review your answers from page 138 in the sequence you ordered them, according to your priorities of the benefits you wish to achieve through regular physical activity.

Please list below your top three answers.

1. _____

2. _____

3. _____

Consider these three benefits to be YOUR primary motivators that will drive your commitment to exercise.

Overcoming Your Negative Exercise Beliefs

"I don't have time. There's too much else to do."

Is it really true that you don't HAVE time? Or is it that you don't MAKE time? I know it sounds clichéd and easy for me to say, but if exercising is that important to you as a means to feeling better and living with greater health, success and happiness, then you can always find a way to make the time. It is all a matter of deciding what is truly important and meaningful to you and your life.

In order to overcome this obstacle in your thinking, I ask that you answer the following questions:

If someone offered to pay you $10,000 per week for the rest of your life, and all you had to do for it was find 30 minutes to exercise five days out of seven each week, given your current schedule of activities and items on your daily To-Do list, do you think you could find the time?

    ❑ Yes

    ❑ No

If you were suddenly diagnosed with a painful life-threatening illness, for which you had to undergo a 30-minute medical treatment five out of seven days a week for the rest of your life in order to survive and live pain-free, would you find the time?

    ❑ Yes

    ❑ No

If someone could guarantee that you would have greater health and happiness with minimized long-term weight-related health risks, and all you had to do for it was find 30 minutes to exercise five days out of seven each week, given your current schedule of activities and items on your daily To-Do list, do you think you could find the time?

    ❑ Yes

    ❑ No

My guess is that you answered *"Yes"* to at least one of these questions. If you answered *"Yes"* to the $10,000 and *"No"* to the health and happiness guarantee, then it clearly reveals that you value money more than your health. My hope is that you answered *"Yes"* to all of the questions. The point is that if there was something in it for you that you deemed valuable enough, then you will find a way to MAKE the time for exercise. The key question then becomes a matter of what you value most. When you make food and life choices that are not conducive to your optimal health and happiness, then you are not living life to the fullest.

All the money in the world can't buy optimal health and happiness. You have to work for it like anything else you want in life.

What do your health and happiness really mean to you?

_____

_____

_____

_____

_____

In my story, I shared how I began by finding a minimum of 30 minutes to exercise a minimum of three days per week. After lots of trial and error, stumbling and getting back on track, I came to the conclusion that working out first thing in the morning works best for me. This may not be the case for you, and that's fine. The key is to find when in your schedule you can make an appointment with yourself for exercise.

Making an Appointment with Yourself to Exercise

When you make a personal, social or work-related appointment, most people will write it in their calendar or agenda, or enter it into their cell phone, blackberry or palm pilot, so as not to forget. I'm asking you to treat your exercise time exactly the same as you would treat any other personal, social or work-related appointment. For those of you who hate routine and lack self-discipline, I ask that you push yourself beyond these self-imposed limitations and give my system a try. I know it works because I still have to do it myself.

I want you to open up whatever system you use for tracking appointments and look at the next six weeks of scheduled appointments. Now I want you to add in all of your usual daily and weekly tasks, activities and responsibilities, no matter how big or small, allotting approximate times you normally spend completing those tasks. If it's outside the house, be sure to account for your travel time there and back as well. For example, if you typically do groceries once a week, then write into your schedule when you do the groceries, how long you're usually there for, and the travel time. If Tuesday night is movie night with your spouse, for example, then I want you to write it into your calendar for the next six weeks. Include the travel time there and back and the approximate time you think you'll be at the theatre. If Thursdays you have to take one of your children to ball practice, then make sure that is all written in the same calendar with everything else. If you watch television after dinner for a few hours, then mark that into your schedule too, with start and end time.

If you're not sure how much time you spend on these activities and when you typically do them, you may want to keep a diary with you at all times for a few weeks, and mark down the start and end time for all your activities. You can then transfer them into your agenda. Over time, you can start to recognize your usual patterns and how you spend your time. You can't be in two places at the same time, so there is no need to keep separate agendas for work, social and personal appointments. I'm asking you to put them all into one agenda so you have the complete picture at hand at any given moment as to your timed activities, tasks and responsibilities.

The idea behind this exercise, which may be more difficult for some of you than others, is for you to become aware of how you manage your time. Here are some questions to consider:

How much time in an average week do you spend on the following activities?

_____ Driving in your car.

_____ Watching television.

_____ Working at your job or career.

_____ Doing chores and running errands.

_____ Socializing with family and friends.

_____ Doing hobbies or other recreational activities.

_____ Preparing meals.

_____ Waiting in lines at fast food restaurants.

_____ Sleeping.

_____ At your computer emailing, surfing the internet, playing games or online chatting.

What else are you spending your time on?

_____

_____

_____

_____

_____

_____

What do you notice about how you are spending your time?

_____

_____

_____

_____

_____

_____

How well do you feel you are managing your time?

_____

_____

_____

_____

_____

_____

If you managed your time better, do you think you could schedule 15 minutes a day, five days a week into your schedule to exercise?

❑ Yes

❑ No

What has to happen in order for you to make it possible to schedule 15 minutes a day, five days a week to exercise?

_____

_____

_____

_____

_____

_____

What are you going to do about it?

_____

_____

_____

_____

_____

_____

When are you going to start?

_____

_____

_____

_____

_____

_____

If you managed your time better, do you think you could find 30 minutes a day, 3-5 days a week to exercise?

❑ Yes

❑ No

What has to happen in order for you to make it possible to schedule 30 minutes a day, 3-5 days a week to exercise?

_____

_____

_____

_____

_____

_____

What are you going to do about it?

_____

_____

_____

_____

_____

_____

When are you going to start?

_____

_____

_____

_____

_____

_____

If you managed your time better, do you think you could find 45 minutes a day, 3-5 days a week to exercise?

❑ Yes

❑ No

What has to happen in order for you to make it possible to schedule 45 minutes a day, 3-5 days a week to exercise?

_____

_____

_____

_____

_____

_____

What are you going to do about it?

_____

_____

_____

_____

_____

_____

When are you going to start?

_____

_____

_____

_____

_____

_____

If you managed your time better, do you think you could find 60 minutes a day, 3-5 days a week to exercise?

❑ Yes

❑ No

What has to happen in order for you to make it possible to schedule 60 minutes a day, 3-5 days a week to exercise?

_____

_____

_____

_____

_____

_____

What are you going to do about it?

_____

_____

_____

_____

_____

When are you going to start?

_____

_____

_____

_____

_____

_____

Let Go of Crippling Attitudes

You'll need to let go of the attitudes discussed in Principle #2 that could interfere with your ability to sustain a reasonable exercise program long enough to see desired results. As you gradually get stronger and better at the exercises, you'll be more and more motivated to push yourself toward even higher goals. However, first you have to give yourself the proper time and chance to see results. It takes time, so give yourself the time you need. What's the rush, anyways?

If you're a perfectionist who thinks in all-or-nothing terms, who feels guilt, shame or self-loathing when you do anything that falls short of your ideal of what perfect is, and if you always put the needs and wants of others ahead of your own, then you have to pay close attention to what I am about to help you with.

Challenging the Need for Perfection

I ask that you start by scheduling only 15 minutes, five days a week into your schedule for the next three weeks. If you're aiming for perfection, and only manage to do 15 minutes on three of those five days, then you'll feel like you have failed. You'll get discouraged and get down on yourself. Instead of getting down on yourself, get your weight down instead, by letting go of this need to be perfect and turn your thinking style into a more positive one. For example, if you manage to get four workouts in week one, five workouts in week two and only three workouts in week three, then just remember you managed to do twelve more workouts than you did in the previous three weeks, and possibly three months or three years, for that matter. Instead of beating yourself up for not getting all five in each week, pay attention to what you did manage to accomplish differently than before, and give yourself a big pat on the back. You should be proud of every success, big or small, perfect or not. After three weeks, add a few minutes and keep adding a few minutes every three weeks till you're doing 30 minutes or more five days a week.

Challenging Your All-or-Nothing Thinking Style

Here's the all-or-nothing trap that your way of thinking may lead you to fall into when it comes to exercise. Let's say you have said to yourself that you would exercise for 30 minutes every evening after dinner for the next five days. You manage to do it the first day and feel great. The next day you're feeling frustrated after a hard day at work and your sister unexpectedly needs you to come baby-sit for her. Now you automatically think to yourself that you can't do your 30-minute workout as planned, so you go to her house and baby-sit and don't do any exercise. Instead, you get the baby to bed and plop onto the couch and watch some television.

After all, you weren't home or couldn't go to the gym, so you couldn't do your workout whether it be a 30-minute walk, pedaling on your exercise bike, lifting weights or whatever it is you intended to do.

I'm going to challenge you on this. Just because your circumstances changed doesn't mean that you couldn't do any exercise at all. You have to learn to get creative and become more flexible and adaptive to unexpected situations. You could have spent 30 minutes in front of the television doing aerobic exercises and lifting weights using soup cans if you had to. Instead of watching television, you could have put on some music and danced for 30 minutes. You could have walked up and down the stairs to get your heart rate up. You could have done something, but in your mind you gave up. You decided that since you couldn't do all of your workout as planned, you would do nothing instead. Perhaps you could keep some portable exercise equipment in your car for just these occasions, such as free weights, exercise bands, a workout video and/or a yoga mat. Even doing stretches would be better than not doing anything at all.

Make a list of the portable exercise equipment you have that you could bring in your car.

_____

_____

_____

_____

_____

_____

If you don't have anything, then what can you come up with that you can buy and have readily available for unforeseen circumstances?

_____

_____

_____

_____

_____

_____

What exercises can you do without equipment?

_____

_____

_____

_____

Let Go of Guilt, Shame and Self-Loathing

Sometimes things will come up unexpectedly that throw you off track. For example, if you're really not feeling well, you hurt your back, or you have a severe migraine, then you have to listen to your body. Your body may need rest or only light stretching more than a strenuous workout that could just be the thing to put you right out. I ask you to use common sense and focus on the big picture. If you have to miss a workout for good reason, then accept your current reality for what it is, and let go of any feelings of guilt, shame or self-loathing. That is, stop beating yourself up when things don't go exactly as planned. Again, getting off track with your workouts doesn't have to mean all-or-nothing. If all you can manage to do is some stretching, then be happy with that. If you hurt your leg, but you can workout your arms, then exercise your arms and whatever else you can, and be happy with that. Just do the best you can in every circumstance, and forgive yourself when you can't make things happen exactly as you'd like them to.

Forget About the Quick Fix Solution

When it comes to working out and getting quick results, you need to be absolutely realistic. Results come over time with gradual building and consistent output of physical effort combined with a healthy eating regime. If you exercise regularly without watching what you eat, you will slow down the results you achieve. If you eat well and only exercise occasionally on a random basis, then you'll also slow down the results. Rather than look for fast results, focus your efforts on finding an exercise regime that you can maintain with consistency long-term.

"I'm too tired." "I have no energy." "I'm too lazy."

Have you ever caught yourself not doing your exercises because you have *"no energy"*, you're *"too tired"* or *"too lazy"*? If yes, then I am here to challenge you yet again. Are you really too tired or too lazy, or is it simply that you THINK you're too tired and/or lazy? The point I'm trying to make is that more often than not, we create our own circumstances by how we think and what we believe to be true. If you keep repeating to yourself in your mind that you're too tired or too lazy to exercise, then you will do whatever is necessary to prove yourself right.

Here is an example. I ask that you imagine yourself in this or a similar scenario, and answer the following questions.

It's Wednesday morning at 6:00 a.m. and you've put into your schedule to exercise for 30 minutes that morning starting at 6:15 a.m. You have planned to do 15 minutes on the treadmill and 15 minutes on the exercise ball followed by some light stretching. You're lying in bed and the moment of truth has come.

You can only choose ONE of the following.

❑ I would get up out of bed and get to it

❑ I would roll over and go back to sleep

If you could realistically see yourself getting out of bed and doing your exercise routine, what is it that made you choose this option? You could have stayed in bed, but you chose not to. Why is that?

_____

_____

_____

_____

If it's more likely that you see yourself rolling over in bed and going back to sleep, what is it that made you choose this option? You could have gotten up out of bed to exercise, but you chose not to. Why is that?

_____

_____

_____

_____

What do you think has to happen for you to CHOOSE to get up out of bed and do your exercises, even in those moments when you might prefer to stay in bed?

_____

_____

_____

_____

_____

_____

_____

Do you remember the self-awareness questions that we used in that moment of truth when you're about to make a food or beverage choice? These questions can be applied to exercise choices just as easily. Here are a series of questions you can ask yourself when about to choose whether or not to exercise.

1) *Why do I want to exercise?*

Look back to your top three benefits/motivators from page 144 for doing regular physical activity, and write them in the space below.

1. _____

2. _____

3. _____

2) *If my long-term healthy weight control and positive living goals are truly as important to me as I say they are, then why would I choose NOT to exercise?*

Possible answers may be any and all of the excuses discussed earlier. Perhaps in this case you are choosing NOT to exercise because you're too tired or too lazy. Perhaps you had a really hard day and just don't FEEL like it. Or you were up playing computer games, reading or out partying till 2:00 a.m. and now just want to stay in bed to get more sleep.

3) *Are any of your reasons NOT to exercise really good enough to choose NOT to?*

❏ Yes

❏ No

Chances are that if you think about your reasons NOT to, compared with all the reasons TO do, then hopefully the reasons to do the exercise will outweigh the reasons not to.

If you decide that your reasons really are not good enough NOT to, then you need to move on to the next question.

4) *Is NOT doing your workout really worth it?*

That is, are the immediate short-term benefits of foregoing the exercise for a little extra sleep, or just doing something else, such as watching television or eating, REALLY worth the cost of your long-term health and weight control goals and desires?

I ask you to forgo what your wants and desires are in the moment, and instead re-focus your thoughts on the bigger picture. You need to get your mind out of the immediate moment and into the future. If you always make your decisions based on what is happening in the moment, you may end up never doing what's best for you in the long-term. You will always find excuses NOT to exercise or eat properly. By always living according to what will give you the most immediate gratification in the present moment, and not remembering the vision for your desired future, you may never reach and maintain your long-term healthy eating, positive living and weight control goals. You need to constantly remember and focus on what it is you truly want for yourself and your life. Your future starts with the decisions you make today, so choose wisely. Choose consciously. Observe your thoughts as if they belonged to someone else, and when you hear those negative self-limiting excuses and beliefs start to infiltrate, I ask you to be strong and push them back. Don't let them in. Challenge them. Overcome them, and replace them with positive thoughts that will propel you to take the actions necessary to turn your desired future into reality. You will be so much happier with yourself every time you do this. It will get easier and easier over time. Just keep at it.

"It's so boring." "It's too hard." "I can never stick to anything."
"I'm not good at anything physical."

Have you ever heard yourself say that you don't exercise because you feel it's too boring, too hard, too tough to stick to, or you're just no good at it? If yes, then don't worry, as you're not the only one. Like many others, you may have come to believe that exercise and physical activity is boring, hard to do, difficult to stick to, and that you're just not that good at it. This is a natural assumption if this is truly your only experience of yourself in relation to exercise and physical activity.

As mentioned previously, I felt this way all through my school years and for much of my adult life. There were always other things that I much preferred doing that came to me much more easily, and that did not require physical exertion. I always felt resistant and resentful toward exercise and physical activity, because I could never accept within myself that it was something that I didn't feel especially good at. It just didn't come naturally to me, so instead, I avoided it at all costs. However, I knew that if I was ever going to be able to embrace physical activity with open arms into my daily life, then something would have to change.

When I started to change my attitude toward food, I remember thinking to myself that food tastes good and that is not going to change. Therefore, the only other part of the equation is ME. I had to change my thinking and behaviour in relation to food. The same is true for exercise. When it came to exercise, I had to stop resisting and simply accept the fact that exercise takes time and consistent effort, and that is not going to change. Therefore, the only other part of the equation is ME. I had to change my thinking and behaviour in relation to exercise. If you struggle with exercise, then the same will be true for you.

To achieve your desired healthy eating, positive living and weight control results long-term, YOU now need to stop resisting reality. YOU are the only part of the food and exercise equation that needs to change. YOU need to change your thinking and behaviour toward exercise. The problem is that to date, in your experience of yourself in relation to exercise, the benefits may never have outweighed the costs of your time and energy. You may have tried getting into an exercise routine in the past, but every time you started and then gave up, for whatever reason or excuse, you felt like an even bigger failure, and became even more convinced that regular exercise just is not for you, and too much work. And so, your conviction that exercise is too boring, too hard and, therefore, impossible to stick to, and that you're just no good at it, became even further entrenched into your belief system and consciousness. And so you continue to struggle, not only with your weight, but with your self-esteem too.

Imagine for a moment what your life would be like if you could let go of these self-limiting beliefs and end the struggle. Imagine, if by letting go, you could actually embrace exercise into your life.

How do you think your life would be different?

_____

_____

_____

_____

_____

_____

What has to happen for you to let go of these self-limiting beliefs?

_____

_____

_____

_____

_____

_____

What is stopping you from making these things happen so you can finally let go of these self-limiting beliefs?

_____

_____

_____

_____

_____

_____

Starting today, what will you do differently to finally let go of these self-limiting beliefs?

_____

_____

_____

_____

_____

_____

"I hate sweating."

This excuse is another classic example of what some people say to themselves to avoid exercise. Is this truly a good enough reason not to exercise at all? Yes, exercise means an output of energy, which creates heat, and leads to sweating. For some people, the thought of sweating makes them feel dirty, uncomfortable or embarrassed. If this is true for you, then the question is, *"What form of exercise can you think of that will lessen the feeling of sweat and perspiration?"* The best solution is aquatic sports. Swimming and water aerobics are excellent forms of exercise and you never have to feel yourself sweating. So this eliminates that excuse. If going to the pool is too much of a bother, then you need to rethink how important your healthy eating, positive living and weight control goals truly are to you. Lots of people will say to me that they don't want to wear a bathing suit in public. I understand that you may feel self-conscious in your appearance, but your options are limited. Either you exercise in the privacy of your own home and potentially work up a sweat, or you do aquatic sports in a bathing suit in public where you won't have to worry about sweating. If you're lucky enough to have a pool in your backyard, then you truly have the best of all worlds. The only problem there, is that you are limited by weather conditions.

"I'm too self-conscious and ashamed of my appearance to work out in public."

I've heard this excuse repeatedly for avoiding exercise completely, and believe me when I say that I have a lot of sympathy for those who feel this way. Worrying about what other people think of you is a hard habit to break. However, one of the greatest gifts you can give yourself is to stop worrying about what others think of you, and just take care of yourself instead. Here are some questions to consider.

How important is it to you what others think of you when you work out in public?

      ❑ It's not important to me at all.

      ❑ It's somewhat important, but it doesn't stop me all the time.

      ❑ It's very important and I will never work out in public.

If it is **somewhat**, or **very important** to you, why do you think that is?

_____

_____

_____

_____

_____

_____

Is this a good enough reason to not do any exercise at all?

      ❑ Yes

      ❑ No

What can you do differently to overcome this obstacle so that you can still manage to incorporate regular exercise into your routine?

_____

_____

_____

_____

_____

_____

What other ways are there to exercise that do not involve working out in public?

_____

_____

_____

_____

_____

Which of these ways are you willing to commit to?

_____

_____

_____

_____

_____

What activities can you do on your own?

_____

_____

_____

_____

_____

How often are you willing to commit to doing these activities?

_____

_____

_____

_____

_____

When will you start doing them?

_____

_____

_____

_____

_____

"I'm afraid of injuring myself." "I have too many physical restrictions."

If these are your reasons for not exercising, then I will challenge you on both counts. Is it really true that you CAN'T exercise because you're afraid of injuring yourself or you feel you have too many physical restrictions, or is it that you CHOOSE not to because of these self-limiting attitudes? Are either of these truly good enough reasons NOT to exercise at all? I have to admit that for a long time I used these exact same reasons (dare I say excuses?). After my car accident in 2003, it took about two years to recover from the injuries I sustained to my back, hip and shoulder. I was given strengthening exercises from the physiotherapist, massage therapist and chiropractor and tried to do them as consistently as possible. However, every time I felt sharp pain, I'd get scared and automatically pull back from doing the exercises. I was so afraid to push myself through the pain, that I let my fears get the better of me. I was also frustrated because I didn't always know how to measure what level of pain was acceptable and okay to continue exercising with, and what level of pain indicated that I should slow down or cut back. It was hard to do any form of cardiovascular exercise because I couldn't stand, walk or do any form of impact aerobic exercise for very long. It took a long time to slowly work my way back to normal.

In looking back, it is easy to see that there were times when I could have pushed a little harder and endured the short-term pain for the long-term gain. I babied myself a bit too much sometimes, which probably made my healing process even slower. I needed to keep moving and do the exercises to strengthen my muscles and ligaments so that the pain would lessen, yet it hurt to do them most of the time, so it was hard to see the light at the end of the tunnel. To this day, I still get flare ups in my lower back and shoulder, and have learned how to take them in stride, and get back on track when they've subsided. I also know what triggers the flare ups and try to avoid these whenever possible.

If you truly do have physical limitations such as a bad back, or neck and shoulder problems, then you are best advised to seek guidance from a trained professional who can give you exercises to lessen these problems, and also exercises you can work on despite these issues. Again, it may not need to be a situation of all-or-nothing. Just because you have some limitations may not necessarily mean you can't do anything at all. You may be restricted in the types of exercise you do, but it doesn't mean you are restricted from everything.

Exercise is often what is needed to alleviate the symptoms of your physical challenges. My mother had a very bad back for as long as I can remember. She ended up with severe osteoarthritis in her spine, which caused her tremendous amounts of pain and grief. I remember when I was a child, her coming home after a doctor's appointment with a list of daily exercises to keep her spine healthy and flexible. I remember her putting a towel on the living room floor and doing her exercises once in a while on a random basis. This lasted for only a short period of time, and eventually she stopped doing them because they caused her discomfort. After seeing how much pain she endured in her later life, I often wondered if the pain would have been as bad had she kept up with the exercises for all those years.

What has happened that makes you so afraid of injuring yourself?

_____

_____

_____

_____

_____

What has to happen for you to overcome this fear?

_____

_____

_____

_____

_____

What will you do about it? What will you do differently?

_____

_____

_____

_____

_____

What is the first thing you will do and when?

_____

_____

_____

_____

_____

"I have nobody to exercise with."

Have you ever heard yourself using this excuse not to exercise? If yes, then I ask you to challenge yourself.

Is it really a good enough reason NOT to exercise?

☐ Yes

☐ No

What is happening that makes it so important to have somebody to exercise with in order to exercise at all?

_____

_____

_____

_____

_____

What would have to change for you to be able to either work out alone, or make more of an effort to find someone to work out with?

_____

_____

_____

_____

_____

What are you going to do about it? What will you do differently?

_____

_____

_____

_____

_____

What is the first thing you will do and when?

_____

_____

_____

_____

_____

Start Slowly

I recommend starting your exercise program gradually. If you're not used to doing regular exercise, I ask that you refrain from putting undue stress and pressure on yourself to do a 30-minute strenuous exercise program right at the start. It will be much safer and more manageable if you ease yourself into the routine. The reason I had you complete some of the earlier questions was to see if you could eventually fit 60 minutes of exercise into your schedule 3-5 times per week. I suggest that even starting with 15 minutes, but committing to doing it 3-5 times per week for a few weeks is a great start and something to be proud of. For the next 3 weeks, I want you to make an appointment with yourself 5 times a week for 15 minutes, where you are totally focused on physical activity. Go for a walk, put on some music and dance, go up and down the stairs, jump up and down, lift some light weights, anything. Just get moving. Be sure to do some light stretches before and more extensive stretching after. Don't get too worried about how hard you work at it quite yet, just get moving and build the habit of taking the time to do it. Don't push yourself too hard at first or you may risk injury. Go easy. With every workout, push yourself just a little bit harder, and with time, you will be amazed at how much you can actually do. If you're feeling winded, dizzy or nauseated, you're probably pushing much too hard, so slow it down. Start slowly with light physical activity and build up to more vigorous activity. You'll want to add up your activities in periods of 10 minutes each and work your way up to being physically active for 30 minutes or more on most (five) days of the week.

Your activities should include a mix that help to build 1) cardiovascular endurance such as aerobics, biking, dancing or swimming, 2) flexibility such as yoga and 3) muscular strength such as lifting weights, water aerobics and other activities that use resistance. Since muscle burns more calories than fat, your aim is to replace body fat with calorie-burning muscle.

IMPORTANT NOTE: *Starting slowly is very safe for most people. However, it is wisest to consult your health professional before beginning any new exercise regime to be sure it is safe for you, especially if you have not been physically active on a regular basis for a long time.*

Here are some ways to incorporate physical activity into your daily routine that all add up at the end of the day:

- Walk whenever possible at a moderate rate.

- Park your car a few minutes walk away from your office or from the store when running errands.

- Instead of going for your usual coffee break, get up and go for a vigorous walk. Go by yourself or find a walking buddy to go with you. If the weather isn't ideal for walking, you can also climb a few flights of stairs to get your heart rate up. This is also a great way to walk off some of the work stress that may be building up in your day. Talking things out with a colleague is also a great way to manage your stress. Your colleague may be able to help you gain a better perspective on your situations and how best to deal with them.

- Keep a set of light weights at your work desk and do some repetitions lifting them with your arms. This will help build strength and flexibility and give you a bit of a mental break as well. If you don't have weights at your desk, then get creative and use something like a couple of full water bottles instead. This is also a good reminder to drink your water.

- Every hour take a few minutes to do some light stretching, especially in the neck, shoulders, upper back, legs and forearms. Forcing your-self to break away from your work and do body stretches can help relieve muscle tension, eye strain at the computer and relieve stress. The next time you're at work feeling anxious or bored, instead of turning to sweets for comfort, break away from your work for a few minutes and do some stretches or go for a walk. Keep away from any snack tables that may be displaying tempting treats.

- When you get home from work, put on your favourite dance music and dance like nobody is watching you for 15 minutes or more. This is a great way to let go of the stresses of the day, energize you and lift your mood. Even if you think you're too tired, put on the music and do it anyway. After a few minutes you just might get into it, if you give it a chance.

- If watching television for long periods, you don't have to be totally inactive. Remember that incorporating activity as much as possible while watching television is also a great way to avoid unnecessary snacking. Try the following:

  • Run on the spot during commercials, instead of reaching for your favourite snack foods.

  • Lift weights on the spot. This is a great way to keep your hands busy so they're not in the snack bowl. It also keeps you busy so you're not heading for the fridge.

  • Take stretch breaks for a few minutes every hour or so to maintain flexibility.

- Play actively with your children or grandchildren. Take them to the park and throw around a Frisbee or ball.

Be sure to change your workouts regularly. People often get stuck in the same exercise routine over long periods of time, and then wonder why they're not seeing results. It is important to remember that your body becomes accustomed to a workout program within 4-6 weeks. You therefore need to make changes regularly to challenge your body, especially since the more fit you become, the less fat and calories your body will burn doing the same level of activity at the same intensity for the same duration. Try different types of cardiovascular workouts such as walking, swimming or dancing, add a couple of longer cardio workouts to your week, change the order of your exercises, or increase the weight and/or repetitions.

Now that you've addressed all of your excuses NOT to exercise, you need to come up with an action plan. Let's see what activities you can do from each of the three areas.

What are five cardiovascular activities you would like to do?

1) _____

2) _____

3) _____

4) _____

5) _____

How often will you do them? _____

For how long will you do them? _____

What time of day will you do them? _____

What days will you do them? _____

What are five flexibility training exercises you would like to try?

1) _____

2) _____

3) _____

4) _____

5) _____

How often will you do them? _____

For how long will you do them? _____

What time of day will you do them? _____

What days will you do them? _____

What are five strength/resistance training exercises you would like to try?

1) _____

2) _____

3) _____

4) _____

5) _____

How often will you do them?   _____

For how long will you do them?   _____

What time of day will you do them? _____

What days will you do them?   _____

Exercise Diary

Just like you're keeping a daily food diary, I ask that you now also use a diary to track your physical activity on a daily basis. In addition to tracking what you did and for how long, I also want you to include your successes and challenges. Perhaps you were really tired and were tempted to forego your workout to watch something on television, but you thought about the short-term gain vs. the long-term pain and chose to do the exercises instead. This would be a tremendous success and one to be very proud of. Perhaps the challenge was to complete the workout once you started because your muscles were a bit sore from the previous workout. Here is a form you can use to track your physical activity.

DAY	ACTIVITY	AMOUNT	SUCCESSES	CHALLENGES

Positive Mental, Emotional and Spiritual Activity

When faced with emotional food triggers that send you reaching out to food for comfort, it's important to first recognize that there are better coping mechanisms that will yield much more positive long-term results. The simple truth is that food is not the answer. This is true not only for your outward appearance, but for your overall health and self-esteem too.

As much as physical activity is part of a healthy lifestyle, so is maintaining a balanced mindset and positive view of yourself and the world around you. Physical activity is one way to relieve some of the pressures that build up with emotional food triggers. Another means to cope with emotions without turning to food is to throw yourself into an activity that distracts your mind from the food focus and obsession. If you have physical limitations, or have already done sufficient exercise for the day, then consider finding activities that you enjoy that don't require tremendous amounts of physical effort.

This means stretching your brain to do things that challenge you, interest you, and lift your spirits with a sense of joy, passion and accomplishment. This could be as simple as doing a crossword puzzle, learning to play a musical instrument, taking a course on something you've never learned before, or going to a seminar. What works for many is to find a creative outlet for their mental and emotional energies. If you've never tried journaling, this is a wonderful way to get your thoughts and feelings out onto paper. I use what I call the *"free flow"* approach. The next time you find yourself turning to food for comfort, instead of eating right away, take a few minutes with a piece of paper and a pen, and write out what you're feeling in that moment, and what you think happened that made you feel that way. Then write about all the reasons you want to shed the weight and keep it off as a reminder, and think of ways to avoid giving in to your unhealthy food trigger. Remember to try and do something differently than you normally would, that you can feel proud of.

Whatever activity you choose to do, it has to be something that you can totally immerse yourself in, where there is no sense of time or space. If you have a hobby or passion, then you probably know what I'm talking about. For example, if you love to play the piano, you may find that you can sit at the piano and practice for a few hours, and yet it may only feel like a few minutes. Or perhaps you like to paint or write, and once you get on a roll and your imagination is leading the way, you know no boundaries. Or maybe you enjoy playing video games, which take you into another zone, where a few hours feel like only a few minutes. I am referring to activities that require thought and focus and keep you in the present moment, where you are not thinking about the past or the future, just concentrating on the task in front of you. It is almost a form of active meditation.

Sometimes the best activity you can choose is non-activity. That is, you may need to completely quiet your mind and not have to think about anything at all. Some examples of these non-activities are taking a hot bath, lying down quietly or simply shutting out the world to close your eyes, breathe deeply and just be.

Any of these activities or non-activities are great to conquer food cravings and triggers because they force you to walk away from the food and put your mind into something else. It is the law of distraction. Distract your mind and body from food when you are looking to eat for no other reason than to comfort yourself, or to give yourself something to do when you're feeling bored or out of sorts.

What are some pleasurable activities you can participate in to distract yourself from food when food triggers hit you, such as boredom, frustration, sadness, loneliness, stress, anxiety, celebration or reward from a particularly good or bad day?

_____

_____

_____

_____

_____

What are some pleasurable non-activities that you can do to quiet your mind and body and just relax completely?

_____

_____

_____

_____

_____

"A" Principle #6:
Assessment

While working on all these elements, you need to constantly assess how you are doing in order to know if what you're doing is in fact working for you or not. You're already keeping a diary for your food intake and exercise. Now you need to measure your results and learn to analyze them. I recommend that you answer the following questions in a daily journal to record your self-reflections. Here are some suggested questions to ask yourself to guide your journal entries.

What did I do differently today that I feel proud of in terms of my eating?

_____

_____

_____

_____

_____

What did I do differently today that I feel proud of in terms of my exercise?

_____

_____

_____

_____

_____

What food triggers or challenges did I face today?

_____

_____

_____

_____

_____

What did I do differently today that I feel proud of in terms of how I dealt with each of these food triggers or challenges?

_____

_____

_____

_____

_____

What challenges did I face today in terms of my eating?

_____

_____

_____

_____

_____

What will I do differently next time to either avoid or overcome these challenges?

_____

_____

_____

_____

_____

What challenges did I face today in terms of my exercise?

_____

_____

_____

_____

_____

What will I do differently next time to avoid or overcome these challenges?

_____

_____

_____

_____

_____

What challenges did I face today in terms of how I dealt with each of my food triggers or issues?

_____

_____

_____

_____

_____

What will I do differently next time to either avoid or better deal with each of these food triggers or challenges?

_____

_____

_____

_____

_____

Here is a sample form you can use to measure your results. I ask that you measure your results no more than once a week. I also recommend that you weigh and measure yourself at the same time of day, since results will vary throughout the day.

TRACKING FORM

STARTING DATE: _____ AGE: _____ HEIGHT: _____

STARTING WEIGHT: _____ STARTING % BODY FAT: _____

DESIRED WEIGHT: _____ DESIRED % BODY FAT: _____

DATE	WEIGHT	% BODY FAT	WAIST/PANTS BELT OR OTHER MEASUREMENT	COMMENTS

"A" Principle #7:
Accountability

If you don't learn how to be accountable to yourself, your likelihood of long-term proper eating, healthy weight management and positive living results is compromised. What I found to be one of my biggest challenges to overcome, was doing it alone. I had nobody to answer to, so I would continuously make the same excuses and mistakes, and feel like an even bigger failure every time I did something I wasn't proud of. I secretly attempted diet after diet, even for only a few days or a week, just desperately wanting to see the numbers go down on the scale. Then, as soon as I stopped the diet, I would see the numbers go right back up. It was totally counterproductive, short-sighted and incredibly disheartening. If I had someone to coach me along and help me discover a better way to eat, feel and live, I could have saved myself a lot of pain and heartache. I could have been a lot happier a lot sooner. However, it is all part of the learning journey. If I hadn't gone through that painful process myself, I would not have been able to fully appreciate and empathize with your challenges as I do now. I can now see my own difficult journey as a gift.

In speaking with professional dieters, I learned that I was not the only one who found it difficult to both reach and sustain my target weight all by myself. I learned that what people wanted and needed above all else was accountability, along with guidance and caring support. This is why I created the 24/7 daily electronic diary system as an integral part of my Healthy Eating, Weight Control and Positive Living counseling practice. What I learned through my clients' experience is how the daily accountability helps them to stay motivated and on track because they know that another human being is listening to them and holding them responsible for their actions.

By making my clients accountable daily, I am forcing them to self-reflect, take ownership of their choices, and be responsible to themselves. I am forcing them to wake up and pay attention to their thinking style and choices. Over time, my clients wean themselves off of being accountable to me and slowly learn to become accountable to themselves by maintaining the accountability habits that they practice while in the program. Accountability can never end. You must always be accountable to yourself. Your choices are yours alone to make. You are responsible for your own decisions, choices, actions and behaviours. When accountability becomes part of your regular mindset, you will be astounded at how it will help you stay motivated, focused and on track. If you let the accountability factor slide, and you get lazy with monitoring your own successes and challenges, you put yourself at risk of falling back into old habits and associated weight gain.

To maintain your proper eating, healthy weight and positive lifestyle, you need to keep accountable for your choices, behaviours and actions for the rest of your life. This is non-negotiable. Even though I have shed my unwanted pounds and continue to keep them off, there is not a day that goes by that I am not fully conscious and accountable to myself for the choices I make. If I choose to over-indulge in a less healthy or high-calorie food choice, I own that choice. I make that choice fully aware and accepting of the consequences. I know how fragile habits can be, and that through self-awareness and accountability, I know I can get right back on track.

How to Create and Maintain Accountability

You can learn to become accountable to yourself on your own as I did. However, what I hear from clients is that it's much easier, especially at first, to have someone outside your regular social circle to be accountable to. This person can be a friend or colleague, but remember that it may be difficult for him or her to be fully objective and honest with you, since there is a close relationship already established. He or she may also not have the food-awareness and professional expertise to give you the level of counseling, coaching and support you need to help you stay motivated and focused, and overcome any bumps in the road along the way.

By seeking the assistance of an outside professional, you get the benefit of total objectivity. This person is not part of your immediate circle of influence, and can therefore be fully objective with you. You can tell this person things going on in your life that may be influencing your emotional eating habits, that you might not even share with your best friend. There is no personal investment in the relationship and confidentiality is respected, so it is safe for you to be as open and honest as you can. The person you are accountable to can help you with your endurance, fortitude, resilience and staying power. He or she can teach you how to eventually become accountable to only yourself. Be sure that whoever you choose to work with is someone who will be an ongoing resource to you.

This is important because as you reach your target weight and work toward maintaining it, you may need an occasional motivational boost when life throws you an unexpected curve ball that derails you from your healthy path. There will undoubtedly be times when your willpower, confidence, courage or steadfastness might wane. You may weaken for a short time, but what will get you back on track is the knowing that you've already done it. You know you can do it, so you can do it again and again no matter what, where or when adversity strikes. However, always be sure to reach out for help if and when you need it. There is no shame in needing outside help and support.

"A" Principle #8:
Appreciation

It's amazing how we're taught to be polite and thankful to others when they do something nice for us or give us a gift, but we so seldom are as polite and thankful toward ourselves. Maybe it has to do with the fact that many of us so seldom truly do something just for us, or give ourselves a gift just *"because"*. How rarely we take the time to truly appreciate our health, our family, our friends, our safety, our home, our food and every other blessing in our lives. It's so easy to take it all for granted. We tend to be so focused on what's missing, what we don't have now, what we wish for, and what we are unhappy and dissatisfied with, that we fail to see the other side of it. We live with a constant cloud hovering over our heads, rather than allow the sun to come shining through.

I ask that you leave those dark clouds behind, and start appreciating the good. Start paying more attention to all the positive efforts and successes you're having each and every day, and learn to acknowledge the challenges, decide how you will deal with them differently next time, and then let them go. If you made a poor food choice yesterday, let it go and just focus on doing better today. If you made a poor food choice a few minutes ago, let it go and start again fresh right NOW. If you're used to having six chocolate chip cookies in a sitting, and today you only had three, then that is a success to be proud of. Recognize the accomplishment of having fewer cookies than you normally would, instead of beating yourself up and feeling guilty over the three that you did eat. It's all about perspective. I ask that you learn how to change your perspective, so that you look at the whole picture and not simply over-magnify your challenges and shortcomings.

When you over-process the problems and challenges in your life, it becomes increasingly difficult and painful, as you may lose sight of the bigger picture. Sometimes it is nearly impossible to see the forest through the trees when you're in a situation without intervention from an outside source. When it comes to your healthy eating, weight control and positive living choices, I ask that you get help when you need it if you can't find anything good to appreciate. Being thankful and able to see the positive side of things, truly is a practice. I ask that you start practicing it right now. When those food triggers hit, I ask that you take a step back and turn your focus away from the food, toward what you are already thankful and appreciative of today, and what you'd be even more thankful and appreciative of in the future.

For example, if you're thankful and appreciative of your current health, in that you don't have any major weight-related health conditions, then imagine how thankful and appreciative you'll be in the future if you can maintain this state of health, or make it even better. When you take an appreciative approach in your thinking, it truly wouldn't make any sense to still go ahead and over-indulge in poor food choices when food triggers hit. Setting your mind on the bigger picture, and getting out of the trap of momentary gratification may help you make the better choice.

What are you thankful for and appreciative of about yourself?

_____

_____

_____

_____

_____

_____

What are you thankful for and appreciative of about your work?

_____

_____

_____

_____

_____

_____

What are you thankful for and appreciative of about your family life?

_____

_____

_____

_____

_____

_____

_____

_____

What else are you thankful for and appreciative of about your life?

_____

_____

_____

_____

_____

_____

_____

_____

Celebration of Successes

To help you appreciate even your smallest successes, it's important to celebrate them by putting yourself up on a pedestal and being kind to yourself. It's all about giving yourself some appreciation for a change. This doesn't mean using food as a reward as you might normally do. It means finding new ways to be kind to yourself without over-indulging in poor food choices or alcohol.

As you start seeing your weight go down, you may want to set mini-benchmarks of either 5 or 10 lbs. That is, for every 5 or 10 lbs you shed (or you can measure by drop in inches or clothes sizes), you treat yourself to something special to make you feel special. Here are some suggestions from what my clients have used to help them celebrate and appreciate their successes and accomplishments:

1) Flowers
2) Massage
3) Perfume/Cologne
4) Pedicure/Manicure
5) Outing to a movie, concert, sporting event or other favourite form of entertainment
6) Music CD
7) Video Game

What else might you like to treat yourself with as a means to celebrate your success?

_____

_____

_____

_____

_____

_____

_____

What will you use as your benchmarks?

_____

_____

_____

_____

_____

_____

_____

How soon after you have reached a benchmark will you treat yourself?

_____

_____

_____

_____

_____

_____

_____

"A" Principle #9:
Acceptance

Acceptance to me means letting go of your attachments to how you believe things are *"supposed"* to be. That is, I ask that you stop resisting what is true and real. I ask that you stop living in an overly idealistic world where you believe that you, others and the world around you should always operate according to how you think they *"should"*, and that things *"should"* be perfect all the time. The fact of the matter is that you are NOT perfect. Others are NOT perfect. The world is NOT perfect. To resist this universal truth will keep you in a constant state of stress. You may continue to try and control others and the world around you as you believe others *"should"* behave and how the world *"should"* operate. I know it is difficult to accept, but in all reality there is very little you have control over. I ask that you consider and accept that the only thing you have control over is YOU. The only thing you can change is YOU.

When you accept reality for what it is, and let go of the need to control everything around you to suit your preferences and what you believe to be *"right"*, or how things *"should"* be, the sooner you will lift a huge weight off your shoulders. The burden of your way of operating in the world is weighing you down. I know, both from personal experience and that of others, that once you lift this burden off of your shoulders, your ability to cope with daily challenges will get stronger and stronger, your stress will be less, and the excess fat you are sick and tired of carrying around will more easily release itself from your body. Once you accept things, it becomes easier to deal with them in healthier ways. Once you are dealing with things in healthier ways, your mind becomes freer and you can focus better on doing what you need to do for YOU, YOUR health and YOUR peace of mind.

I am not suggesting here that you accept the unacceptable. For example, if you are being physically or verbally abused by your partner, I am not suggesting that you accept this behaviour. I am simply suggesting that you see the reality of your situation. If you have been in denial, then I ask that you accept reality. Once you accept the truth of your reality, then you are in a better position to take action and do something about it.

Accepting Compliments from Others

I remember when I started trimming down, people giving me compliments about how great I looked, especially if they hadn't seen me in a long time. I can still remember the first time a male friend told me I was looking *"hot"*. The word *"hot"* was not a word I had ever associated with who I was or how I saw myself. It definitely did not fit the image I had of myself and my body. *"Was I really hot?"*, I wondered quietly to myself. As you can imagine, I felt rather awkward and bewildered at first at such a compliment.

I was used to thinking of myself as someone who was overweight and could stand to shed a few pounds. But now I was no longer overweight. Therefore, the story that I had on myself for so long no longer held true for me. It was strange at first, as I had to change my image or belief of who I was in my outward appearance. I had to let go of the Roslyn who saw herself as overweight and out of shape, who dreaded shopping for new clothes, who felt embarrassed and ashamed of her body in a bathing suit, who avoided sexy, tight fitting clothes so as not to feel self-conscious, who lacked confidence in her ability to control her eating, embrace physical activity, manage stress and balance her life. It took some time to mentally adjust to the new physical me. As I adjusted, it became easier to accept compliments from others. With time, it actually made me feel really good, and I learned to simply say *"Thank you"* rather than get embarrassed and try to say things to negate the compliment. I needed to learn and accept that it was okay to feel proud of my accomplishment. You too, should feel proud of your self-change and achievement. You worked hard to get where you are. Of course people are going to notice, and I ask that you accept any sincere compliments with utmost honour and grace.

Accepting the New *"YOU"*

At the same time I was trying to adjust to receiving compliments I wasn't used to getting, I had to both accept and embrace the new me. The new Roslyn was now in good shape and a healthy weight. As a result, she could shop for new clothes much more easily, and no longer felt embarrassed and ashamed to be seen in public wearing a bathing suit, or self-conscious wearing sexier and more form-fitting clothes. She finally had the newfound confidence that she could control her eating, exercise regularly, and better balance her life. The new Roslyn felt great.

As the weight came off slowly, my clothes started to fit looser and looser, especially my pants. Rather than buy new clothes, I brought my clothes to the seamstress to be made smaller. I remember the first time I bought a brand new pair of pants once my healthy weight was stabilized. I had no idea what my new size was. I used to wear a size 14, sometimes 16, so I thought that I must at least be down to a size 9 or 10. I tried on a series of pants in size 10 and, to my amazement, they were ALL too BIG. I couldn't believe it. I couldn't remember a time I was ever less than a size 10. I then tried on a new series of pants in size 8. Some fit perfectly, and some were still too big. Overwhelmed with emotion, I found myself crying in the store's fitting room. Putting on size 6 pants and feeling great about how they fit, was a wonderfully surreal experience.

The funny thing is that eighteen years ago, which is probably the last time I weighed what I weigh today, I was not a size 6 or 8. What this tells me is that at age forty, I must carry my weight quite differently than I did at twenty-two. I remember weighing 120 lbs when I was in high school and wearing a size 9 or 10 jeans. If I weighed 120 lbs today, I would be too thin. This goes to show how insignificant the number on the scale really is. Being a realistic healthy weight doesn't necessarily mean weighing what you did when you were sixteen or eighteen. Your body changes over the years, so I ask that you accept your healthy weight as being the weight that makes you look and feel great at the age you are today. There is no need to be too thin. Having a few extra pounds is not necessarily a bad thing. I always think that if I ever got sick again, at least I have flesh on my bones to fight with.

I shared this story with a client of mine part way through her program with me. She experienced something similar when, after losing 62 lbs, she went on a trip and decided to try on a two-piece bathing suit. She was absolutely thrilled and chose to buy it. Buying a bikini and feeling great about how she looked and felt in it was symbolic that she had finally arrived. She worked hard on changing her lifestyle and reprogramming her relationship with food, and her inner and outer self. She deserved to feel proud of herself, as you will too, when you do what you need to in order to eat better, feel better and live better.

Accepting Others

As you develop healthier eating habits, get into shape and live a more positive, balanced life, you will start to become more aware of how others around you are eating, and choosing to live their life. That may or may not change as you change. It is important to remember that just because you are choosing to change your ways, does not mean that others will necessarily follow suit. Your spouse, partner, friends and family did not go on your journey, you did. They may continue to eat, drink and live as they always have. You may be tempted to preach to others by telling them what they should eat and how much, to get more active or better balance their lives. You may be tempted to get them on The A List program, but this kind of preaching can be damaging to your relationships, as others may resent you for it, and secretly wish you would just leave them alone. They may have no desire to change. They may not be ready. If, however, they repeatedly complain about their eating habits, weight issues or life problems, or tell you how much they admire you for your accomplishments, *then* you may want to encourage them and give them support. You may then want to ask if they truly want to change their life. If they say *"yes"*, then you may want to tell them about the **9 "A" principles** and encourage them to take the first step.

Others may give you a hard time when you muster up the courage to say *"no"* to dessert, or take only a small serving instead of your usual portion. They may say you're no fun. They may give you a hard time when you choose not to put heaping portions of food on your plate like you used to. They may give you a hard time when you take less alcohol. They may make comments or poke fun, or instead, they may tell you how much they admire you for being so strong and taking such good care of yourself. I ask that you not concern yourself with negative comments from others. They too, have to accept the new YOU, just like you do. They have to learn to accept your new ways. If they have trouble doing so, then that is for them to resolve and not you. If they continuously try to sabotage your efforts or break down your resolve, then you have to ask yourself what kind of friends they really are, as this is very disrespectful. Just as you have to respect their food and lifestyle choices, even when they've just finished telling you how unhappy they are with their weight, they must respect you and your choices in your efforts to take good care of yourself. I ask that you not let others stop you from keeping up your good habits. If necessary, you may need to sit them down and explain how important this is to you, that their support would be greatly appreciated, and then spell out exactly what you need from them in the way of support.

Accepting Attention

As you gain confidence in your appearance and feel better about yourself, you'll find yourself walking with an extra bounce in your step, more energy and more enthusiasm. You may not realize it, but you will actually start to shine and radiate to others. Your positive energy will be undeniable, and people will notice. You may get more looks from the opposite sex. You'll have to learn how you manage this newfound attention, especially if you're not used to it. Your spouse or partner may have to get used to it too. It is your job to decide what you want to do with that newfound attention.

I once had a client who struggled with her weight for years. I asked her my usual question *"Is there any reason you can think of to keep the weight on?"* Her answer was very telling. After giving it some thought she stated the following:

"When I was slim, I used to get a lot of attention from men. I really liked it. But now that I'm with my husband I'm afraid of what will happen if I shed the weight and start getting all that attention again." I asked what exactly she was afraid of. She said *"I'm afraid I won't be able to trust myself."* This statement was crucial to her long-term success, because unless she addressed this underlying issue, she would continue to fail at every weight management attempt. She will continue to self-sabotage even her best efforts because she's not truly prepared to shed her excess weight for fear of the possible consequences that she has already built up in her mind.

The reason I'm sharing this story with you is because you will have to always remember what is truly meaningful and important to you. Having newfound confidence includes having the confidence in your ability to manage yourself appropriately and not take the increased attention you might get from the opposite sex any farther than it needs to go. You must be very clear on your boundaries of what are acceptable and unacceptable behaviours.

Conclusion

There is no doubt that we live in a fast-paced, ever-changing world that can keep us trapped like a rat on a spinning wheel, but only if we continue to allow it to. The problem is many of us don't feel like we have a choice. We just continue spinning our wheels, and don't even stop to realize how it is impacting our overall health, happiness and quality of life. The only way to stop this cycle is by recognizing and reconnecting to what is truly meaningful and important in our lives. We have to stop trying to operate like machines, and instead reconnect to all that makes us human.

As we have seen, a large part of what keeps us spinning are our habits, beliefs and attitudes toward ourselves, others and the world around us. For any long-lasting life change, including how we eat, how we feel and how we choose to live our lives, we need to recognize, challenge and conquer our unhealthy and counterproductive habits, beliefs and attitudes that continue to keep us in a negative relationship with food and our inner selves. We have to start looking after ourselves better and making our health a top priority in our lives. We may believe ourselves to be programmed as the perfectionist, people pleaser, rescuer and nurturer who prefers to avoid conflict and never be a burden on others. We may be wired to want to always appear nice and unselfish due to a strong need to be liked and admired, but we have to look at how all these ways in which we've been programmed are affecting our emotional health. When these attitudes start to take their toll on our physical, mental, emotional and spiritual well-being, then we have to take notice and take a stand to strike a better balance, or we will end up in a perpetual state of unhappiness.

My sincerest wish for you is that you will embrace the perspectives, information, insights and tools in this book, and put them into daily practice. I ask that you review the questions that you answered. Come back to them every few months, and see how your answers may have changed. Use them to help you self-reflect and come to understand yourself better. Remember that if you need, or simply want, outside help, don't be afraid to ask, and always seek professional help.

My biggest hope is that you will finally let go of how you believe things were *"supposed"* to be, accept what your true reality is today, and then do what you need to do to create the life you want for your tomorrows. I invite you to share this book with others and welcome your feedback and comments on how this book has helped you change your life.

Send comments to **info@roslynfranken.com**

Recipes

Roslyn's Fast and Easy Beans and Couscous

This recipe can be used as a side dish or main course. Because it combines a starch with beans, it actually forms a complete protein. It can be served hot or cold. You can prepare a large amount ahead of time, and then bring leftovers for your lunch the next day. It is also a great snack in-between meals. It is highly nutritious, high in fibre, low in fat, low in calories, and combines foods from four of the six main food groups including grain, vegetable, meat and healthy fat. The only things missing are the dairy and fruit. You can always top off the meal with some yogurt with fruit and, presto, you've covered all your food groups. It's also very easy and fast to prepare. You can experiment with different ingredients according to your tastes and also play with different spice combinations for a nice variety in flavours. Instead of beans, you can use diced, cooked leftover skinless chicken or turkey. You can even try it with canned tuna or salmon.

2/3	cup uncooked couscous
2/3	cup boiling water
1	onion chopped
4	cloves garlic crushed
3	cups of your favourite mixed chopped vegetables such as broccoli, red, green, yellow or orange peppers, cauliflower, carrots, celery, tomato. You can use fresh or frozen.
1	can of your favourite beans such as kidney, romano, black beans, lentils or chick peas
¼	cup feta cheese crumbled (optional)
2	tbsp olive oil
1	lemon
2	tsp dried basil
1	tsp oregano

Place couscous in a large bowl with tight fitting lid, or have a large plate ready to cover the bowl with.

Boil water in kettle.

When water has boiled, pour over the couscous and cover tightly, with either the lid or plate. Let stand for 5 minutes minimum.

While letting couscous stand, combine chopped onion with raw chopped vegetables and sauté in frying pan with a little bit of cooking spray. If using frozen, mixed vegetables instead of fresh, then cook according to instructions. To save time you can:

- Chop the vegetables the day before and have them ready in the fridge.

- Buy a vegetable platter from the grocery store where the vegetables are already pre-cut. This is more expensive but a great time saver.

- Use frozen mixed vegetables instead.

When vegetables are tender crisp, add beans and seasoning and mix well till heated through. By this time the couscous should be ready.

Uncover couscous and fluff with a fork. Add sautéed vegetables and beans and mix well.

Add olive oil and lemon juice.

Garnish with crumbled feta cheese.

VARIATIONS – Don't be afraid to get creative.

For a more Indian flavour, try seasoning with some curry and cumin to taste and add ¼ cup of raisins. Or, add a little bit of Indian chutney according to taste. It's great with mango chutney.

For a more Mexican or Tex-Mex flavour, stir in some Salsa or BBQ sauce.

For a more Asian flavour, stir in some low sodium soy sauce or sugar-reduced spare-rib sauce.

Roslyn's Quick and Easy Chicken Recipes
Doesn't Get Faster Than This!

These recipes shouldn't take you longer than 5 minutes to prepare and an hour to cook. I suggest making them in larger quantities so that you can freeze leftovers for quick lunches and dinners. The beauty of these recipes is that you can use the chicken in different ways. You can unfreeze leftovers and make a chicken salad, cut it up and mix it with rice, add it to a soup, or slice it up for a quick sandwich with mustard, lettuce and tomato on whole wheat bread.

Barbecue Chicken

Enough boneless, skinless chicken breasts, or your other favourite chicken parts with skin and excess fat removed, to cover bottom of baking dish.

¼ cup Barbecue sauce per chicken serving

Preheat oven to 350 degrees Fahrenheit.

Line a large glass baking dish with aluminum foil for quick and easy clean up. Spray with cooking spray. This will prevent the chicken from sticking to the foil.

Place skinless, boneless chicken breasts, or your favourite chicken parts with skin removed, in the large glass baking dish.

Pour your favourite BBQ sauce over the chicken and ensure the chicken is well covered with the sauce.

Cover the baking dish with aluminum foil and place in preheated oven.

Bake for 1 hour.

Allow to fully cool before freezing leftovers.

Avoid eating extra sauce as it will have the fat in it from the cooked chicken. This means **do not** pour the sauce over your rice or other side dishes, and **do not** pour extra sauce over your chicken. The chicken should have enough sauce on it when you remove it from the baking dish for flavour.

VARIATIONS – *Instead of BBQ sauce, use Salsa.*

Pineapple Chicken

Preheat oven to 350 degrees Fahrenheit.

Line a large glass baking dish with aluminum foil for quick and easy clean up. Spray with cooking spray. This will prevent the chicken from sticking to the foil.

Place skinless boneless chicken breasts or your favourite chicken parts with skin removed in the large glass baking dish.

1	cup tomato ketchup
1	16 oz can of pineapple chunks with liquid drained
1	tsp powdered ginger
1	chopped onion (if you have the time)
1	chopped green pepper (if you have the time)

Combine all ingredients in a medium bowl. Pour over chicken. Cover the baking dish with aluminum foil and place in preheated oven. Bake for 1 hour. Allow to fully cool before freezing leftovers.

Roslyn's Mexican Bean Spread

Here is a great healthy, low-fat, low-calorie and easy to prepare alternative to the usual fatty cream and cheese dips and spreads that pack on the calories. It's best served as an appetizer with tortilla chips, pita bread or cut up raw vegetables. It's a great dish to bring to your next potluck or BBQ as well. You can also use it as a sandwich spread.

1½	cups canned kidney beans drained and rinsed
3	tbsp water
1	tbsp tomato paste
1	tbsp lemon juice
1	tsp ground cumin
¾	tsp dried oregano, crumbled
¼	tsp hot red pepper sauce (optional)
Pinch	ground cinnamon

Using a food processor or blender, blend the kidney beans, water, tomato paste, lemon juice, cumin, oregano, red pepper sauce, and cinnamon for 1 minute or until smooth.

Makes 1½ cups.

Roslyn's Sweet Potato Peanut Butter Soup

This soup is filling, nutritious and low in calories. It includes a number of spices that are excellent for digestion with antioxidant properties. You can experiment with different amounts, or omit spices that you aren't fond of. It also contains garlic and ginger which have many healthful qualities as well. If you aren't as crazy about garlic as I am, try putting in less. Start your meal with a bowl of this soup, or use it as a snack when you need a little something to fill you up.

1	sweet potato cubed
2	onions diced
1	tbsp light tasting olive oil
1	carton 900mL reduced sodium, fat-free chicken broth
4	cloves garlic crushed
1	tsp curry
½	tsp turmeric
½	tsp black pepper
½	tsp cumin
½	tsp coriander
28	oz can of crushed tomatoes (low sodium if possible)
2	tsp finely grated fresh ginger
2	tbsp light peanut butter

Boil the sweet potato till tender, about 15-20 minutes. Drain. Mash potatoes, add the grated ginger, and stir well. Put aside.

In a large pot, heat the oil on medium high heat and fry the onions and garlic till softened.

Add the curry, turmeric, pepper, cumin and coriander and stir for 1 minute.

Add the chicken broth and crushed tomatoes and stir. Allow to boil.

Add sweet potato and ginger mixture and peanut butter. Turn heat to low and allow to simmer for 20 minutes.

Freeze leftovers in individual serving size containers for quick additions to your lunches or for snacks.

For more recipes, please visit **www.roslynfranken.com**

Do you have a healthy recipe you'd like to share?

Send it to **info@roslynfranken.com**

Information Sources
that have influenced my writing:

Amen, Daniel G., M.D., Change Your Brain, Change Your Life, Time Books, New York,1999.

Gillespie Larrian, The Menopause Diet, Healthy Life Publications, Beverly Hills, 2002.

Heart and Stroke Foundation of Canada Website, www.heartandstroke.ca

Plutt, Mary Jo, Prevention's Stop Dieting & Lose Weight Cookbook: Featuring the Seven-Step-Get-Slim Plan That Really Works, Rodale Press Inc., New York, 1994.

Reivich, Karen, PhD & Andrew Shatte, PhD, The Resilience Factor: 7 Keys to Finding Your Inner Strength and Overcoming Life's Hurdles, Broadway Books, New York, 2003.

Sarno John, M.D., The Mindbody Prescription, Warner Books, New York, 1999.

Science Daily Website, www.sciencedaily.com

Whitney, Eleanor Noss, Understanding Nutrition, Thomson Nelson, Scarborough, 2004.

About the Author

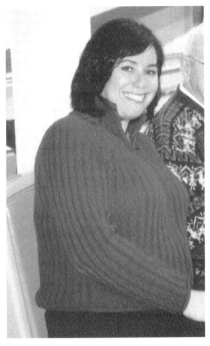

BEFORE

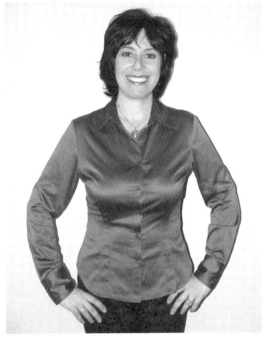

TODAY

Diagnosed with cancer at age twenty-nine, Roslyn Franken fought back to become a long-term survivor. The experience provoked her return to school (Masters in Human Systems Intervention from Concordia University in Montreal and certification through the Professional School of Psychology in California) and inspired a career as a counselor, personal coach and motivational speaker.

As she approached forty, Roslyn's personal struggles with her weight led to the creation of the techniques that changed her life. By putting the principles into practice, she reached and maintains her current, healthy weight and remains cancer-free. Roslyn now primarily counsels clients who want to change their lives for the better through healthy eating and positive living, using the insights she developed and now shares in *The A List's* 9 principles.

Roslyn is happily married to Elliott, a professional magician, and enjoys portraiture, the healing arts, cooking, and song writing.

The **A** List

by Roslyn Franken

For information on booking the author for speaking engagements and personal counseling, or to purchase copies of this book, please visit www.roslynfranken.com or call toll-free 1.877.852.5852 or 613.843.0155

Register today for Roslyn Franken's FREE Healthy Hints Online Newsletter at www.roslynfranken.com